# KETO DIET FOR WOMEN OVER 50

# 4 in 1

## Dr. Leanne Axe

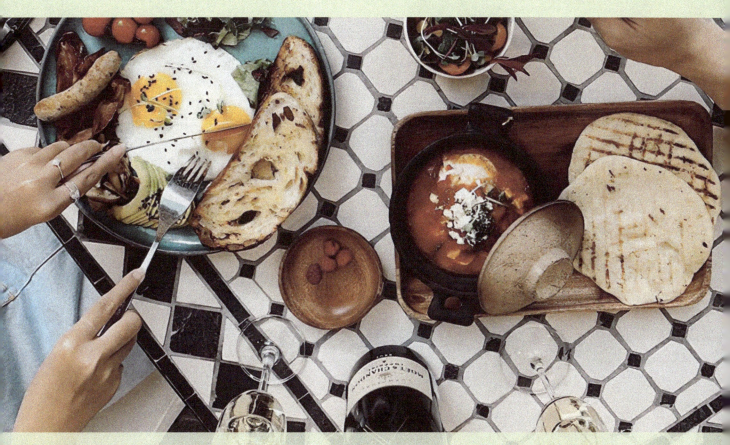

A HealthYou Book

New York

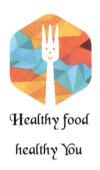

SIRTFOOD DIET

2020 © Copyright by Dr. Leanne Axe

Use of any content by Dr. Leanne Axe is prohibited except with written permission from the publisher.

The Author is not engaged in rendering professional advice or services to the individual reader. The ideas, procedures, and suggestions contained in this book are not intended as a substitute for consulting with your physician. All matters regarding your health require medical supervision. The Author shall not be liable or responsible for any loss or damage allegedly arising from any information or suggestion in this book.

While the Author has made every effort to provide accurate researches, numbers and other information at the time of publication, she does not assume any responsibility for errors or inaccuracies. Further, the Author does not have any control over and does not assume any responsibility for third-party websites or their content.

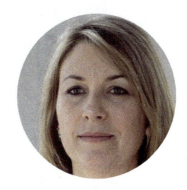

To my beloved hubby Jack and my two little creatures.

"If you keep good food in your fridge, you will eat good food."

Errick McAdams

"An optimist is a person who starts a new diet on Thanksgiving Day."

Irv Kupcinet

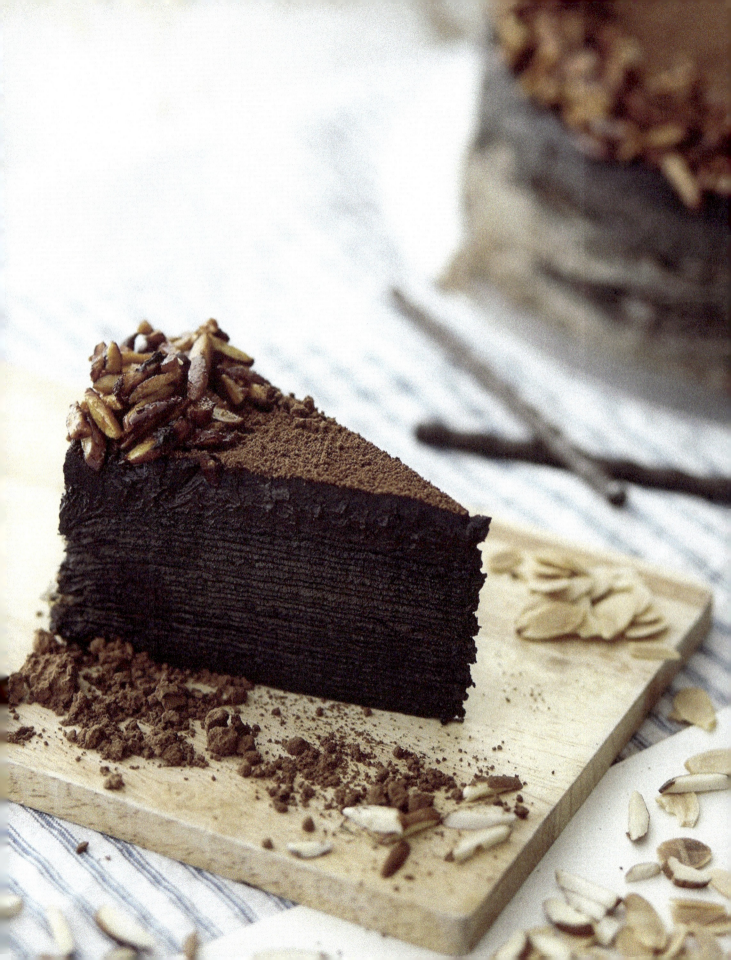

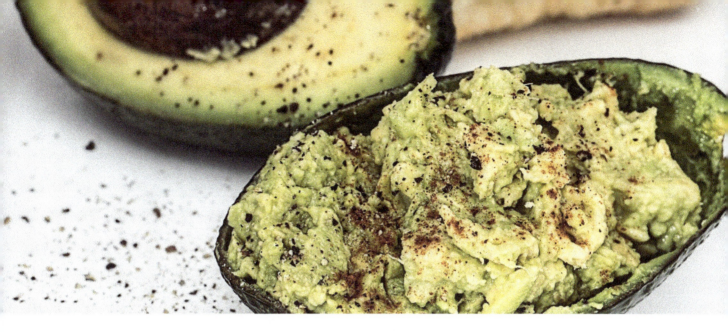

## Table of Contents

| | |
|---|---|
| **The Author** | 1 |
| **Introduction** | 3 |
|   Obesity Epidemic | 3 |
| **Part 1** | 8 |
| **The Ketogenic Diet, explained** | 8 |
| **Chapter 1: What is a Keto Diet** | 9 |
| **Chapter 2: The Pros and Cons of a Keto Diet for Women Over 50** | 13 |
|   Advantages of the Keto Diet for Postmenopausal Women | 14 |
|     Improved Health | 14 |
|     Energy & Mental Performance | 14 |
|     A Healthier Stomach | 15 |
|     Increment Insulin Sensibility | 15 |
|     Prevent Weight Gain | 16 |
|     Stimulate Weight Loss | 16 |
|     Helps Fight Cravings | 17 |
|     Potential Cancer Treatment | 17 |
|     Drastic Reduction of Triglycerides | 18 |
|     Treatment of Parkinson's Disease | 18 |
|     Treatment of Migraine Headaches | 18 |
|   Disadvantages of the Keto Diet | 19 |
|     Potential Side Effects | 19 |
| **Chapter 3: The Ultimate Keto Diet Food List** | 23 |
|   Foods to Eat and to Avoid | 23 |
|   Foods to Eat | 23 |
|     Meat and Protein | 23 |
|     Fats and Oil | 24 |

- Fruits for Keto diet ............................................................................................................... 25
- Keto Veggies ........................................................................................................................ 25
- Dairy for Keto ...................................................................................................................... 26
- Keto Nuts ............................................................................................................................. 27
- Keto Sweeteners .................................................................................................................. 28
- Keto Drinks .......................................................................................................................... 28

Foods to Avoid ............................................................................................................................. 29
- Whole Grain ........................................................................................................................ 29
- Fruits .................................................................................................................................... 29
- Veggies, Legumes & Beans ................................................................................................ 30
- Dairy Items .......................................................................................................................... 30
- Meat ..................................................................................................................................... 31
- Oils and Other Bad Fats ..................................................................................................... 31
- Alcohol ................................................................................................................................. 31

# YOUR JOURNEY STARTS RIGHT HERE ........................................................................... 39
# SCIENTIFIC REFERENCES ................................................................................................... 40
# PART 2 ........................................................................................................................................ 42
# KETO DIET RECIPES ............................................................................................................... 42
# BREAKFAST RECIPES ............................................................................................................. 43

- JILL'S CHEESE-CRUSTED OMELETTE .......................................................................... 44
- CLASSIC BACON AND EGGS ......................................................................................... 45
- SCRAMBLED EGGS ........................................................................................................... 46
- EGG BUTTER WITH SMOKED SALMON AND AVOCADO ..................................... 47
- OMELET WRAP WITH SALMON & AVOCADO ......................................................... 48
- SULLIVAN'S DOUGH BREAKFAST PIZZA ................................................................... 49
- PANCAKES WITH BERRIES AND WHIPPED CREAM ............................................... 50
- FRITTATA WITH FRESH SPINACH ................................................................................ 51
- MUSHROOM AND CHEESE FRITTATA ........................................................................ 52
- ALL DAY KETO BREAKFAST ........................................................................................... 53
- BREAKFAST SANDWICH ................................................................................................. 54
- KETO CORNBREAD ........................................................................................................... 55
- TOMATO BAKED EGGS ................................................................................................... 56
- CHOCOLATE PANCAKE CEREAL .................................................................................. 57
- EASY BANANA MUFFINS ................................................................................................ 58
- CHICKEN CURRY PIE ........................................................................................................ 60

# MAIN MEALS ............................................................................................................................. 60

- BUFFALO DRUMSTICKS WITH CHILI AIOLI ............................................................... 62
- CHICKEN WINGS WITH CREAMY BROCCOLI ........................................................... 63
- PEPPER-CRUSTED BEEF TENDERLOIN WITH HERBED STEAK SAUCE ............... 64
- MEXICAN CAULIFLOWER RICE ..................................................................................... 65
- TACO PIE .............................................................................................................................. 66

| | |
|---|---|
| POT BARBECUE CHICKEN | 67 |
| SPAGHETTI SQUASH CASSEROLE | 69 |
| JALAPENO POPPER CHICKEN CASSEROLE | 70 |
| KETO STIR FRY | 71 |
| CRISPY LEMON BAKED CHICKEN THIGHS | 72 |
| PESTO CHICKEN CASSEROLE WITH FETA CHEESE AND OLIVES | 73 |
| STUFFED CHICKEN BREAST WITH ZOODLES AND TOMATO SAUCE | 74 |
| CREAMY CHICKEN, BACON AND CAULIFLOWER BAKE | 75 |
| CAULIFLOWER MASH | 76 |
| EASY TOFU PAD THAI | 77 |
| CRACK CHICKEN | 78 |
| NO NOODLE LASAGNA | 79 |
| GINGER LIME CHICKEN | 80 |
| BRESAOLA PLATE | 81 |
| TURKEY WITH CREAM-CHEESE SAUCE | 82 |
| PIMIENTO CHEESE MEATBALLS | 83 |
| GOAT CHEESEBURGER WITH ZUCCHINI FRIES | 84 |
| HAMBURGER PATTIES WITH CREAMY TOMATO SAUCE AND FRIED CABBAGE | 85 |
| OVEN-BAKED PAPRIKA CHICKEN WITH RUTABAGA | 86 |
| CARAMELIZED ONION AND BACON PORK CHOPS | 87 |
| TEX-MEX CASSEROLE | 88 |
| CHICKEN GARAM MASALA | 89 |
| SKILLET PIZZA | 90 |
| CELERY & BLUE CHEESE SOUP | 91 |
| THAI FISH CURRY | 92 |
| CHICKEN ALFREDO | 93 |
| EASY SWEDISH MEATBALLS | 94 |
| EASY CHICKEN CHOW MEIN | 95 |
| **KETO SNACKS** | **96** |
| STUFFED & GRILLED VEGETABLE BITES | 97 |
| ULTIMATE GUACAMOLE | 98 |
| AVOCADO WITH TAMARI & GINGER DRESSING | 99 |
| CHEESY AUTUMN MUSHROOMS | 100 |
| KETO SNACK BOX | 101 |
| MEXICAN EGG ROLL | 102 |
| CAULIFLOWER TOTS | 103 |
| SALAMI CHIPS | 104 |
| PROTEIN BALLS | 105 |
| BACON BUTTER | 106 |
| GARLIC BREAD | 107 |
| KETO SALAD | 108 |

**DESSERTS** .................................................................................................................. 109
    FRAPPUCCINO SLICE ............................................................................. 110
    CHOC-ORANGE BLISS BALLS ................................................................ 111
    KETO BOUNTY BARS .............................................................................. 112
    CHOCOLATE CHIP COOKIE FAT BOMBS ............................................. 113
    CHOCOLATE PEANUT BUTTER PROTEIN BARS ................................. 114
    CHOCOLATE MOUSSE ............................................................................ 116
    CHOCOLATE CHAFFLE RECIPE ............................................................ 117
    CHEESECAKE FLUFF .............................................................................. 118
    PUMPKIN PANCAKES ............................................................................. 119
    FRENCH TOAST CASSEROLE ................................................................ 120
    FUNFETTI COOKIE BITES ...................................................................... 121
    BLACKBERRY CHEESECAKE ................................................................. 122
    STRAWBERRY CHEESECAKE ................................................................ 123

**PART 3** ........................................................................................................... 124

**30-Day Keto Diet Meal Plan** ........................................................................ 124

**PART 4** ........................................................................................................... 131

**The Keto Diet Journal** ................................................................................. 131

**Final Words** ................................................................................................... 167

# The Author

Dr. Leanne Axe is a seasoned veteran dietitian-nutritionist who herself struggled for many years with her weight before reaching a turning point in her life. One day she decided to take charge of her life... and change it for good.

Now, through her guides, she is changing millions of others'. The author of the best-seller book "Keto For Women Over 50" has been living this lifestyle since 2016. This shift allowed her to lose over 80 lbs. Leanne graduated from the Institute of Integrative Nutrition's Health Coach Training Program.

She earned a Doctor of Education degree in Gifted and Talented Education (2007), a Master's degree in Natural Sciences (1995), and a Bachelor's degree in Elementary Education (1990). Her story has been inspiring women and men of all ages.

The author's declared purpose is to make people "the best version of themselves." Her business has grown throughout the years, but her focus on making people healthier has always remained consistent. She is here to help people lose weight, identify food sensitivities, and improve nutrition through proper meal plans.

Furthermore, Leanne is a passionate cook, so rest assured you will always find mouth-watering recipes when purchasing one of her books.

# Introduction

## Obesity Epidemic

As indicated by the most recent studies, the average citizen in America is getting fatter! Since the 1960s, the obesity rate of Americans has quadrupled! At the moment of writing, the estimates tell us that 25% of American adults are overweight, while an alarming 18% of American kids are getting fatter and fatter. Such percentages repeat more or less in the same way all around the world, especially in industrialized countries.

It is essential to reverse the impacts of obesity on our society.

Overweight people are highly exposed to coronary illness, diabetes, tumors, bone and joint issues, and several other medical conditions. Were we, as a society, to put more efforts into diminishing the percentage of obese individuals in the population, this could also result in cuts in health expenditure.

While french fries, pizza, and franks might be delicious, they assist you with shedding pounds and living longer in no way. If you need to get in shape for personal or medical reasons, you must adhere to an eating regimen that includes a wide range of organic products, vegetables, and whole grains. Every one of these foods will provide your body with the essential minerals and vitamins it needs to function properly.

Generally, not only do foods grown on the ground give you minerals and other precious nutrients, but they are also low in calories, letting you eat bigger bites without putting on weight.

## Introduction

Moreover, whole grains are a big ally to staying healthy and fit. After all, they contain a lot of fiber, a nutrient that will make you feel full for longer.

As obvious as it may seem, a healthy eating routine is the least expensive type of medication one could ever purchase. Smart diets– namely, eating protocols including organic and healthy foods, – are the first, yet the most important, step to gradually get through the obesity epidemic.

People around the world choose various foods for various reasons. Eating with wellbeing in mind is only one of the factors behind the food choices we make each day. Actually, there are specific explanations behind picking one food over another, such as moral and ecological reasons. Other people follow a specific regimen due to food hypersensitivities, allergies, or other clinical conditions. Ultimately, we have our own ideas about what nourishments we need and which we do not.

A few people imagine that if their eating regimen works for them, everybody should eat their way. This is somewhat determined by one's conviction that a specific way of eating is superior to another.

As trivial as it may sound, there is no one-size-fits-all way to deal with smart dieting. Notwithstanding, some fundamental rules are generally recommended and accepted by the scientific community.

In a globalized and varied world as the one we are living in at the time of writing, there are several more or less popular diets to choose among, including:

- Plant-based diet
- Mediterranean diet
- Low-fat diet
- High protein diet

## How is Keto Different from Other Diets?

## Introduction

The ketogenic diet, or "keto diet," is a type of a low-starch diet based on a low-carb/sugar consumption with the declared purpose of putting the body into a state called "ketosis."

Ketosis is that process in which the body utilizes fat (instead of carbs) as its primary source of energy. As we will see in more depth later, whole grains, fruits, legumes, most dairy, and starchy vegetables are among the foods you will skip out on.

So, are you ready to begin your journey to weight loss and massive health? Let us get started!A Successful Weight Loss Story

*with Jessica Megan, one of my beloved patients*

"I've been dissatisfied with my weight ever since I can remember. Back in September 2017, I saw a picture that had been taken of my family and me... then I fully realized how sad and fat I looked. In those years I had been experiencing depression, I had pulled back from social situations, and I was almost hopeless. I felt like at that point I hit rock bottom and decided I was unable to take it any longer. At that time, my weight had reached a record-breaking number: 283 pounds [128 kg]. I avoided having pictures of me taken and started missing out on building memories with my husband and children. Anyway, something positive happened: I decided the time had come to take care of myself and get back in shape."

What were the most significant changes you made to lose weight?

"Firstly, I know I needed to re-instruct myself on how to eat properly. After reading your book, I started following the keto diet protocol.

The first stage was pretty though. Anyway, I knew I needed to radically change the way I thought about getting back in shape. There is no particular secret; it's all about exercising and eating the right foods. It's not just about looks; it's about my wellbeing, too. I need to be

## Introduction

*healthy for my children and husband, and I want to influence them with my new healthy choices."*

What was the most challenging thing about losing weight?

*"Overcoming my fear of eliminating the pleasure of eating. I have struggled a lot in understanding what to eat, when to eat, and the right amount to eat. Then I found the first edition of this guide. It sounded simple, yet it turned out to be a journey. A journey that takes devotion and responsibility. But once you have started, you are basically halfway."*

When did you start to get (and see) results?

*"Actually, I began getting results pretty fast, I would say in the first two weeks. For the first month, I recorded all that I ate in the Sirtfood Journal you gave me and exercised for 30 minutes per day, 6 days every week. I shed 11 pounds [5 kg] in the first 14 days. And now, after 2 years, I am 120 pounds off and finally satisfied with my weight."*

What do you think of your current weight?

*"I could not be happier. It took me 2 years to get to my final weight goal. I realized that slower is better. Losing weight gradually implies you're making the right choices. I haven't taken any diet supplements or similar. I just exercised and ate foods low in carbs and higher in fat."*

How do you manage to keep your weight off?

*"I'm actually still slowly losing weight at this point. I keep on recording what I eat because I think that this motivates me to stay in control of my weight. I believe discipline is a key factor. Now I know that my body needs it, and also my mind and my heart."*

How has your life changed since you've lost weight?

*"My life has changed a lot. I used to be discouraged, I would cry, and I was so miserable all the time. Now, I feel fabulous! I smile more, I get more things done, and spend more quality*

## Introduction

*time with my family. From time to time I still feel the way I used to feel back then, and I wouldn't exchange anything for it. I would never come back to be that disastrous person I used to be."*

How do you think this book will help the readers to achieve their weight loss goals?

*"This 4 in 1 guide will definitely help women over 50 know more about the ketogenic diet, they will learn what to eat, and how to put everything into practice, for a real change of life. And to top it off, the journal will be a strong motivator for their journey! I believe information is power, the more you know, the more you learn, the happier you are. And readers will definitely love the information they will get from this book.*

# PART 1

## The Ketogenic Diet, explained

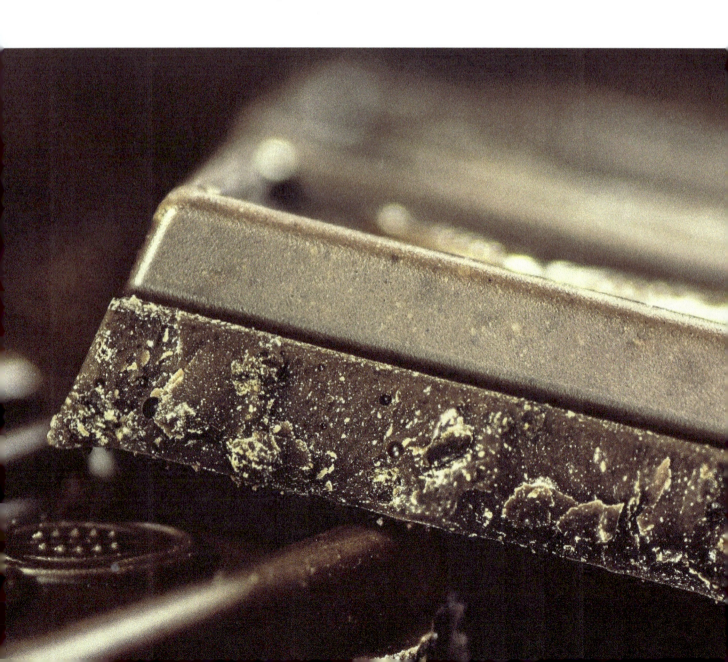

# Chapter 1: What is a Keto Diet

The ketogenic diet (keto diet for short) is a low carb and high-fat eating routine that shares lots of its concepts with Atkins and other low carb diets.

Being on a keto diet means a critical decrease in your sugar admission, which will be replaced with fat. As discussed in the introduction, this reduction in sugars places your body in a metabolic state called *ketosis*.

Once this occurs, your body will be exceptionally effective at consuming fat for energy. In such a state, your body will automatically transform fat into ketones (highly efficient energy molecules) present in the liver, which give power to your body and mind.

The keto diet causes a strong drop in glucose and insulin levels. This has several medical advantages, as we will discover later.

Types of Ketogenic Diet

There are a few variations of the ketogenic diet, including:

Standard ketogenic diet (SKD): characterized by low-sugar, medium-protein, and high-fat food consumption. Generally: 70% fat, 20% protein, and just 10% sugar (percentages could slightly vary, based on your medical condition and weight goals).

Cyclical ketogenic diet (CKD): this includes a period in which you have a higher sugar consumption; for example, 5 standard ketogenic days followed by 2 high-starch days. Weight lifters or competitors usually use this kind of eating protocol.

Targeted Ketogenic Diet (TKD): here, you consume sugars only for more intense workouts to facilitate recovery.

High-protein ketogenic diet: this is like the standard ketogenic diet but includes a higher protein consumption. The proportion is generally: 60% fat, 35% protein, and 5% starch.

*Note to the reader: the data presented in this book apply to the Standard Ketogenic Diet (SKD).*

History and Beginning

In 1921, the pioneering researcher in diabetes and nutrition Russell Wilder prescribed a low-carb diet to treat refractory epilepsy, introducing the name "ketogenic diet." Indeed, at first, this diet was recommended in the clinical field as a healing diet for kids with epilepsy until it knew a period of disuse during the '40s and '50s.

Nevertheless, following the ketogenic diet as a quick weight reduction protocol is a moderately new idea that has proved to be exceptionally successful.

A Little Bit of Biochemistry

Sugars are the principal fuel source in our body tissues. When the body lacks sufficient sugars because of reduced consumption (less than 25 g per day in adults with normal Body Mass Index - BMI), insulin release diminishes as well, taking our body from an anabolic state (where the body builds and repairs muscle tissue) to a catabolic state (where the body loses overall mass, both fat, and muscle).

Stores of glycogen (a polysaccharide of glucose that serves as a form of energy storage) provide the power to our body for any metabolic activity. Two metabolic cycles occur when sugars are low in the tissues of our body: glucose creation and ketogenesis. When the glucose introduced with the foods strongly diminishes, internal glucose creation is not enough to handle the body normal functions, and ketogenesis starts to supply a different source of energy in the form of chemicals called ketones.

In other words, ketones replace glucose as the primary energy source. In ketogenesis, because of low glycemic control, the release of insulin decreases, reducing fat and glucose storage as a result. In this condition, the liver quickly metabolizes fatty acids into molecules named Acetyl-CoA; some of these molecules are then converted into ketone bodies: *acetoacetate*, *beta-hydroxybutyrate*, and *acetone*, which function as both signaling molecules and energy sources. It is important to note that ketone bodies are created with no adjustment in blood ph.

The condition we just discussed is totally different from *ketoacidosis*, a dangerous situation where ketone bodies are created at a rate that is too quickly, converting the pH of the blood into an acid state. This is caused by a deficiency of insulin in type 1 diabetes or late-stage type 2 diabetes.

Ketone bodies, when properly created, are effectively utilized for energy by the heart, muscle tissue, and kidneys. They provide an exceptional energy source for the mind, too.

The body's creation of ketones relies upon a few factors, for example:

Basal metabolic rate (BMR),

Body mass index (BMI) and

Muscle Versus Fat Ratio.

Ketone bodies produce an organic combination named adenosine triphosphate (ATP - a chemical that stores and releases energy for many cellular processes) more than they make glucose. Think that 100 grams of acetoacetate produce 9400 grams of ATP, and 100 grams of beta-hydroxybutyrate generates 10,500 grams of ATP; instead, 100 grams of glucose creates just 8700 grams of ATP. This permits the body to continue producing fuel, even during a calorie deficiency.

# Chapter 2: The Pros and Cons of a Keto Diet for Women Over 50

Since you bought this guide, you might be keen on getting back to the shape you had in your 30s. Well, you are in good hands!

At the age of 50+, numerous women experience a change in their digestive system, particularly a slower digestion, which can cause food to move slowly through the colon.

Add to this less exercise, muscle loss, and the tendency to have more cravings: you will have the perfect recipes to gain weight (or, at least, to make it hard to control it).

While nowadays there are many eating regimes to get back in shape, the keto diet is one of the most popular, mainly due to its effectiveness.

## Menopause

Menopause is a physiological cycle in women characterized by the end of periods and the impossibility of getting pregnant naturally. This is mainly caused by a gradual decline in female regenerative hormones and can be accompanied by symptoms such as:

- Flushing
- Sleep issues
- Night sweats
- Vaginal dryness
- Urinary incontinence
- Reduced interest in sex
- Irritated skin

Research showed that changing your eating routine is an effective way to help balance hormone levels and therefore reduce the abovementioned effects of menopause.

Let's now look into more depth at how the ketogenic diet can specifically affect postmenopausal women.

## Advantages of the Keto Diet for Postmenopausal Women

### Improved Health

Many studies show that a rich-in-carbohydrates diet increases the number of significant risk factors for heart disease, including high-density lipoprotein (HDL) cholesterol and triglycerides. Cholesterol and LDL (low-density lipoprotein) levels are usually moderately affected. It is frequent to see a rise in blood sugar & pressure and insulin levels, though. These consequences are generally associated with the so-called *"metabolic syndrome,"* an insulin-resistant condition that increases your risk of heart disease, stroke, and type 2 diabetes. Such conditions can be prevented thanks to a low-carb diet.

### Energy & Mental Performance

Many people choose to go on a ketogenic diet to improve their mental performance.

Our brain normally needs glucose to function since some parts of it can only burn this kind of sugar. In keto, the brain does not require carbohydrates from food. On the contrary, it is continuously stimulated by ketones, together with some glucose produced by your liver to make up for a very low carb intake.

As discussed earlier, this mechanism has been used for several years to treat epilepsy in kids who don't respond to drug treatment.

For mature women, ketosis causes a constant flow of energy to the brain, avoiding problems such as high blood sugar fluctuations. Thus you will have more focus, get rid of brain fog (you avoid feeling like a nap in the afternoon), with a resulting improved mental clarity.

Keto diet is also correlated to an improvement in Alzheimer's Disease symptoms. Plaques and tangles characterize this form of dementia in the brain that affects memory. It is interesting to note that it shares features of both epilepsy and type 2 diabetes, such as the inability of the brain to use glucose or inflammation related to insulin resistance. A controlled study on 140 people with AD who started a keto diet showed improvements in mental function for 54% of the group.

## A *Healthier Stomach*

The keto diet can "silence" your stomach noises: less gas, fewer spasms, and less irritation that can also result in an overall improvement in IBS (Irritable Bowel Syndrome) symptoms.

For certain individuals, this is one of the biggest advantages; it regularly takes just a day or two for your stomach to become acclimated to this keto diet's benefit.

## *Increment Insulin Sensibility*

Since menopause can cause several changes in hormone levels, for example, modifying the degrees of sex hormones (such as estrogen and progesterone), it reduces insulin sensibility too. This can interfere with the body's ability to utilize insulin successfully.

Insulin is a hormone responsible for moving sugar from the circulatory system to your cells, where it is used as an energy source. Studies have indicated that a ketogenic diet can improve insulin sensibility for better glucose control. One research carried out in 1934 found that insulin sensibility in ladies with endometrial or ovarian cancers was positively affected after a 12-week ketogenic diet.

Nonetheless, it is still not clear whether the keto diet would give comparable advantages to menopausal women without this sort of disease.

Different studies report that reducing starches can lower insulin levels and fix hormonal discrepancies that are particularly frequent during menopause.

Furthermore, researches show that insulin reduction might be related to a higher risk of hot flushes.

## Prevent Weight Gain

As you already learned, weight gain is a typical manifestation of menopause in women over 50 because it is linked to changing hormone levels and slower digestion. While clear evidence on the ketogenic diet is still limited, a few investigations have demonstrated that reducing starch admission help prevent the weight gain related to menopause.

A 2002 study on 88,000 postmenopausal women indicated that a low-sugar diet was linked to a decreased risk of weight gain. Interestingly, the low-fat eating routines were correlated to a higher risk of weight gain. Note that the low-sugar diet used for this research included a higher amount of starches compared to the standard ketogenic diet.

## Stimulate Weight Loss

Strictly linked to the previous one, this is most likely the #1 advantage you bought this guide for. As a matter of fact, the keto diet promotes weight loss by boosting your metabolism and reducing your appetite as well (thanks to the reduction of hunger-stimulating hormones.) In a 2009 meta-analysis of 11 different randomized controlled trials, researchers proved that women over 50 on ketogenic diets lost 7 lb. (3.2 kg) more than ladies on low-fat diets during a 1-year timeframe.

## Helps Fight Cravings

It's common that women experience cravings while menopause progresses. This is because mature women's brains generally have an increased brain reward system activation.

Anticipating food consumption leads to cravings for food and a decreased reward system activation during actual food intake, which induce overeating.

Gut-derived hormones, such as glucagon-like peptide-1 (GLP-1), are involved in the regulation of food intake. As shown by research conducted in 2001 on 205 women in their sixties, the ketogenic diet helps regulate the amount of GLP-1. Similarly, another study noticed that a ketogenic diet diminishes the levels of ghrelin, a hormone that stimulates cravings. In the near future, more investigations are likely expected to assess how the ketogenic diet can influence cravings in menopausal women.

## Potential Cancer Treatment

Based on the assumption that all living cells feed on sugar (also cancer cells eat glucose - blood sugar), some researchers affirm that glucose reduction experienced on a keto diet is directly linked to a reduced risk of cancers in mature women. Some experts believe that the keto diet may be particularly beneficial for brain and breast cancers. A low-carb diet can certainly help when used alongside traditional treatments. Anyway, more randomized clinical tests are needed to correlate sugar in the diet and cancers. Still, for a large part of the scientific community, this benefit remains a myth.

## Drastic Reduction of Triglycerides

Triglycerides (fat molecules circulating in your bloodstream) are the main heart disease risk factor. In elderly people, even the simple sugar fructose may drive elevated triglycerides. One of the contributory causes is a sedentary or less active lifestyle, typical in women around 65-70. A study published in the prestigious journal PubMed showed that carbohydrate restriction leads to a dramatic reduction in blood triglycerides. On the contrary, low-fat diets usually cause them to increase.

## Treatment of Parkinson's Disease

Parkinson's Disease is a nervous system disorder caused by a low level of dopamine, a signaling molecule. This condition often results in tremors, stiffness, and difficulty walking. As seen earlier, the keto diet proved to have protective effects on the brain; thus, it has been prescribed as a complementary therapy for PD. In a 2001 randomized study, 12 women out of 22 following the standard ketogenic diet over 6 weeks showed a 41% improvement in symptoms. Still, this area needs further research.

## Treatment of Migraine Headaches

Generally, as you get older, you will experience a natural improvement in migraine headaches (if you used to suffer from this condition when younger), since hormonal factors now play a minor role. Still, the number of women with migraine in later life is significant. According to some researches dated back to 1928, the keto diet causes an improvement in migraine frequency and severity. Many studies have been carried out on this particular field: for example, a 1936 randomized controlled study proved that 21% of women following a keto diet experienced no migraine attacks for up to 2 months, while another 17% reported a reduced frequency. Later on, this medical application knew a period of disinterest due to the introduction of over-the-counter drugs for managing the condition. Other researchers have instead linked the reduction of migraine symptoms to weight loss more than to the keto diet itself.

As seen above, several health conditions may benefit from a ketogenic diet, such as:

- Obesity
- Metabolic syndrome
- Glycogen storage disease
- Diabetes
- Some cancers
- Alzheimer's Disease
- Migraine

These huge benefits clearly explain the massive popularity keto diets have and why you should absolutely try it, especially if you are a woman over 50.

After exploring the benefits of the keto diet, you will probably also want to know about the side effects so as to decide if this diet protocol is right for you.

## Disadvantages of the Keto Diet

### *Potential Side Effects*

A few studies have connected the keto diet with an increase of LDL (bad cholesterol) and endothelial dysfunctions, a type of coronary artery disease in which there are no heart artery blockages. In a randomized study conducted in 2009 on 1,000 ladies in their 70s who followed a ketogenic diet for 3 weeks, a 39% increase in LDL was shown.

In another controlled study on the dietary benefit of the ketogenic diet, members didn't meet the suggested daily intake of calcium, folic acid, magnesium, potassium, thiamine, and vitamins D and E.

Also, some studies have proved that individuals on a ketogenic diet ingest less fiber than people on low-fat diets.

However, the abovementioned side effects occur mainly when people drastically reduce carb consumption without any professional advice (DIY keto diets).

Another known side effect of the ketogenic diet is the so-called *keto flu*, a condition you could experience when your body enters into ketosis. While your body is switching from using sugar as a source of energy to using your body's fat, you may feel not so great at first and experience temporary symptoms, such as:

- Weakness
- Irritability
- Constipation
- Nausea
- Vomiting
- Headache

In the process of breaking down fat, the body creates ketones that are later expelled through frequent urination, which lead to an inevitable loss of electrolytes (such as sodium, magnesium, and potassium) and can intensify these symptoms. Anyway, you should think of this phase as an adjustment stage. Consider that for most women, the keto flu only lasts about 5-7 days.

The loss of electrolytes discussed above could also lead to kidney stones, mainly due to dehydration. Luckily, there is a simple, natural way to effectively prevent them: stay hydrated. Try to drink around 8 glasses of fluids daily. Obviously, this number should be increased if you work out or sweat a lot. If you do not feel like drinking water, lemonade is an excellent alternative. The trick to telling if you are drinking enough is to look at the color of your urine: it should be clear or pale yellow. Another precious tip, if you have keto flu or a headache, is to add a sprinkle of salt to your glass of water (you should do this especially in the first days, while your body is adjusting to the new changes).

Based on my experience as a nutritionist, the keto diet can result challenging for some women to stick to and lead to yo-yo dieting, causing other negative effects on health. Don't fret! You are in good hands. Later on in this guide, you will find two powerful tools that have already proved to be effective for hundreds of patients and now will assist you through your journey: The Keto Diet Meal Plan and Journal!

*N.B. Always consult your physician before beginning any diet.*

# Chapter 3: The Ultimate Keto Diet Food List

## Foods to Eat and to Avoid

Perhaps the hardest part when beginning the keto diet is understanding which foods are the best to introduce into your diet. Don't worry, though — not only are keto foods mouth-watering, but they also can keep you full and satisfied. Let us discover what foods to eat and what to avoid to help your body enter ketosis!

As you know by now, keto foods have a strictly limited amount of carbs; they're moderate in protein and high in fat. The dietary macronutrients are divided into around 55% to 60% fat, 30% to 35% protein and 5% to 10% carbs. Looks complicated? At the end of this chapter, you will also find a complete list of foods so that it will be easy for you to write down your shopping list to look at when you're at the grocery store.

## Foods to Eat

### *Meat and Protein*

You should eat protein at a moderate level: only about one-fifth of your diet. My piece of advice is to try to buy meat from non-intensive farms (such as grass-fed beef), as this will reduce your intake of steroid hormones and microbes. Skinless chicken should be eaten sparingly, while the grilled chicken is a keto-friendly option. Eggs and oily fish are another great protein source allowed in your keto diet. Oily fish, in particular, are rich in omega-3 polyunsaturated fatty acids, which have been shown to reduce inflammation and lower the risk of heart disease, cancer, and arthritis.

Steaks are another great source of protein. Here my piece of advice is the thicker the cut, the better. Thus: ribeye and sirloin steaks are ideal for keto!

## Fats and Oil

Since your fats form around 60% of your macros, it is vital to understand which ones to consume. The best are those that originate from natural sources like meat, nuts, sunflower seeds, and avocado. Other monounsaturated fats such as olive and coconut oils are fundamental for your keto diet.

As a general rule, you should be cautious with polyunsaturated fat. Stay away from trans-fat, no matter what. Despite these are naturally found in milk (not keto-friendly because of its high carb count), they are often synthetically added to packaged foods, such as snacks and baked goods. Those fats have been connected to coronary illness and elevated cholesterol.

Here's a brief list of healthy fats you should consume (*you will find the complete list at the end*):

- Egg yolk
- Fatty fish
- Ghee
- Olive oil
- Coconut oil
- Nut oil
- Butter
- Mayonnaise (avoid those high in sugar or other carbs)
- Cocoa butter

## Fruits for Keto diet

Luckily, some fruits are low in carbs and thus perfect to be consumed within a keto diet regimen. Moreover, fruits contain fiber, an indigestible kind of carbohydrate that you do not have to count in your daily carb count!

Avocados are the symbol of the keto diet and, as a matter of fact, they are the best organic products you can eat. While you should avoid high-carb natural fruits like bananas, you are still allowed to consume strawberries and watermelon, for example.

## Keto Veggies

Vegetables should constitute a great deal of food in your diet. They are rich in vitamins, minerals, fiber, and phytonutrients. Anyway, not all veggies can be part of a balanced keto meal plan for an important reason: some of them are high in carbs.

Take sweet potatoes. You love them, right? Well, they are loaded with vitamin A and C, fiber, and other phytonutrients. However, 100g (3.5 oz.) contains around 20 grams of carbs! On the other hand, one cup of raw spinach only contains 1g of carbs.

Most vegetables grown on the ground are keto-friendly. Check out this brief list:

- Romaine lettuce
- Swiss chard
- Celery
- Radish
- Cauliflower
- Eggplant
- Cucumber
- Cabbage
- Green beans

- Broccoli
- Kale
- Bell peppers
- Tomatoes

## Dairy for Keto

If you are a dairy lover, you by now have probably realized this simple equation:

dairy = sugars = carbs

Dairy products are such great sources of protein, potassium, fat, calcium… that it would make no sense to completely eliminate them from your diet.

"So, can I eat dairy or not?"

The solution is to consume the lowest carb dairy products (0-3 grams per 100 g/3.5 oz.), such as:

- Butter
- Ghee
- Soft-ripened cheese (Velvety Brie, Camembert)
- Aged cheese (cheddar, Swiss, provolone)
- Semi-soft cheese (mozzarella, Montenery Kack, Havarti)
- Plain Greek yogurt
- Heavy whipping cream

You can moderately consume middle carbs dairy products, such as feta and parmesan cheese, light and sour cream, cottage cheese, kefir, ricotta cheese, or whole-milk plain yogurt. These foods contain 4-7 grams of carbs per 100 g/3.5 oz.

## Keto Nuts

Nuts and seeds have amazing nutrition profiles. Obviously, not all of them are keto-friendly. Once again, you want to consume the ones with the lowest amount of carbs per serving.

They can be eaten as a snack between meals, toasted and tossed into salads, or ground into butter to spread on veggies or low-carb crackers.

Keto-friendly options are:

- Brazil nuts
- Pine nuts
- Macadamia nuts
- Hazelnuts
- Walnuts
- Almonds
- Pecans

Anyway, you have to be cautious when consuming nuts. They contain many fats, calories and thus are very nutritious, but you should keep in mind that they are ok only if you need extra energy; otherwise, you will be only introducing unnecessary calories and fat.

<u>Minimizing snacks should be the rule if your goal is to lose weight</u>. A trick is to consume non-salty nuts. In fact, adding salt to nuts makes them almost addictive. I also recommend avoiding munching nuts while in front of the TV, reading, or doing another activity that catches your attention.

To sum up, if you are hungry and need energy: consume nuts. If you want to lose weight, eating nuts could slow down the process.

## Keto Sweeteners

Probably you were wondering, "Oh, *will I ever be able to add sweeteners to my favorite foods?*" Fortunately, there are some very low-carb sweeteners that have shown to have little impact on insulin levels, including:

- Stevia
- Allulose
- Xylitol
- Erythritol
- Monk fruit extract

## Keto Drinks

Water, either still or sparkling, is simply wonderful (and your body needs it). However, it is not the only beverage you can have on a keto diet!

We already discussed the importance of staying hydrated. When you are out with family or friends, or even when you simply fancy drink something different, you can consume dark espresso or tea. These are magnificent keto-friendly energizers and help with weight reduction, too. Some people on keto love to prepare the Bullet-proof espresso (BPC), a rich and creamy coffee filled with grass-fed butter (MCT oil) and black coffee. It is the perfect fuel to get you moving in the mornings.

Contrarily to other eating regimes, moderate consumption of some specific types of alcohol is allowed on the keto diet, such as:

- Gin
- Vodka
- Whiskey
- Rum

- Pinot noir
- Merlot
- Low carb beers

## Foods to Avoid

### *Whole Grain*

The problem with whole grains, as you could imagine, is simple: they contain sugars. These foods hinder the process of ketosis and should therefore be avoided (or, at least, consumed in very limited quantities):

- Oatmeal
- Rice
- Wheat Grains
- Whole Wheat Flour
- Barley
- Rye
- Quinoa
- Corn

### *Fruits*

We have already seen that avocado, strawberries, and olives are a must to consume since these are high in nutrients and rich in healthy fats. Most fruits are high in carbs, making the following avoidable if you are on a keto diet:

- Pears
- Grapes
- Apples

- Mangoes
- Peaches
- Apricots
- Apples

## Veggies, Legumes & Beans

The keto rule says to stay away from vegetables grown beneath the ground (starchy veggies) since they usually are high in carbs.

Legumes and beans, typically high in nutrients like iron, zinc, and potassium, with good protein content, are high in carbs, too.

- Avoid:
- Peas
- Corn
- Potatoes and sweet potatoes
- Artichoke
- Beans (Black, Baked, Green, Lima)
- Lentils

## Dairy Items

While not all dairy products are banished from the keto diet, you should always avoid highest carb dairy foods(12-25 grams of carbs per cup), including condensed milk, buttermilk, sweetened or fruit-flavored yogurt, or light yogurt. Be sure to read labels before buying, as some products marketed as "light" contain added sugar instead.

## Meat

Avoid, among others, meat with added carbs, such as bacon with added sugars, breaded meat, and other processed meats that may contain concealed sugars. Once again, you should be careful when buying and always read the label.

## Oils and Other Bad Fats

Contrary to what you would think, vegetable oils are not healthy fat sources. Actually, research showed that they can be linked to obesity, type 2 diabetes, and heart disease. Moreover, vegetable oils are rich in omega-6 fatty acids, contain a high amount of polyunsaturated fats and partially or fully hydrogenated oils, which can produce negative effects on your health.

Avoid corn, canola, cottonseed, grapeseed oils; you can still consume the high-oleic variety of safflower and sunflower oils, but keep in mind that the regular variety of these two is not good for keto.

*Pro tips*: when cooking, keep oil below its smoking point (check it on the label) and when heating oil, bring it up to the right temperature slowly; always store oils in a cool, dark location (light and heat damage oil).

## Alcohol

Most commercial beverages are rich in sugars. Stay away from:

Commercial beer (contains an average of 13g of carbs per can)

Cocktails (has up to 46.67g per glass!)

Wine coolers (with an average of 14g per glass)

Sangria (an average of 19.2g per glass)

# FOODS TO EAT

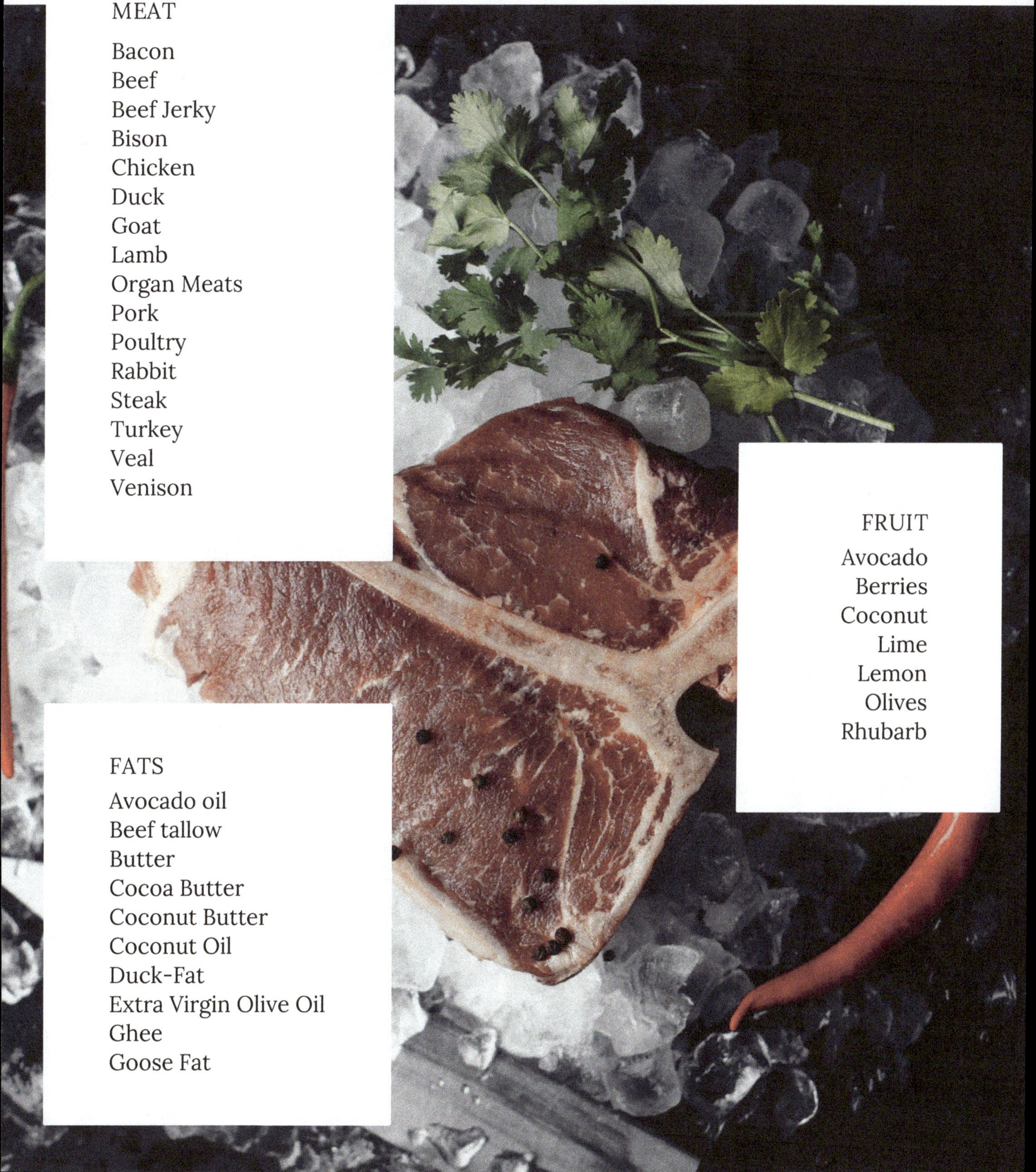

MEAT

Bacon
Beef
Beef Jerky
Bison
Chicken
Duck
Goat
Lamb
Organ Meats
Pork
Poultry
Rabbit
Steak
Turkey
Veal
Venison

FRUIT

Avocado
Berries
Coconut
Lime
Lemon
Olives
Rhubarb

FATS

Avocado oil
Beef tallow
Butter
Cocoa Butter
Coconut Butter
Coconut Oil
Duck-Fat
Extra Virgin Olive Oil
Ghee
Goose Fat

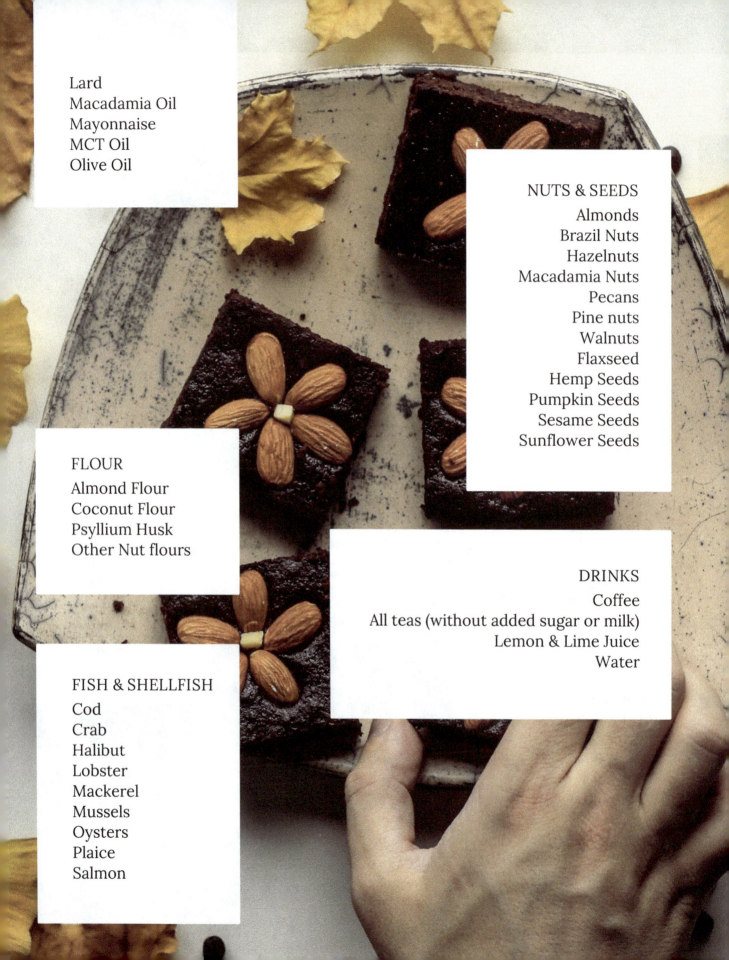

Lard
Macadamia Oil
Mayonnaise
MCT Oil
Olive Oil

### NUTS & SEEDS
Almonds
Brazil Nuts
Hazelnuts
Macadamia Nuts
Pecans
Pine nuts
Walnuts
Flaxseed
Hemp Seeds
Pumpkin Seeds
Sesame Seeds
Sunflower Seeds

### FLOUR
Almond Flour
Coconut Flour
Psyllium Husk
Other Nut flours

### DRINKS
Coffee
All teas (without added sugar or milk)
Lemon & Lime Juice
Water

### FISH & SHELLFISH
Cod
Crab
Halibut
Lobster
Mackerel
Mussels
Oysters
Plaice
Salmon

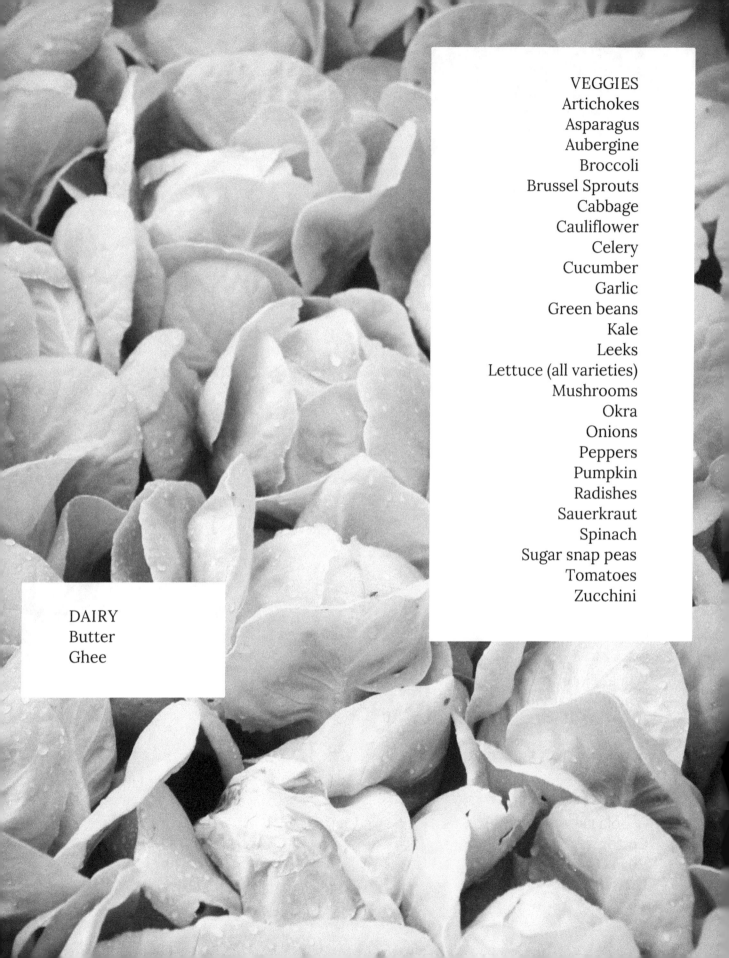

## VEGGIES
Artichokes
Asparagus
Aubergine
Broccoli
Brussel Sprouts
Cabbage
Cauliflower
Celery
Cucumber
Garlic
Green beans
Kale
Leeks
Lettuce (all varieties)
Mushrooms
Okra
Onions
Peppers
Pumpkin
Radishes
Sauerkraut
Spinach
Sugar snap peas
Tomatoes
Zucchini

## DAIRY
Butter
Ghee

# FOODS TO AVOID

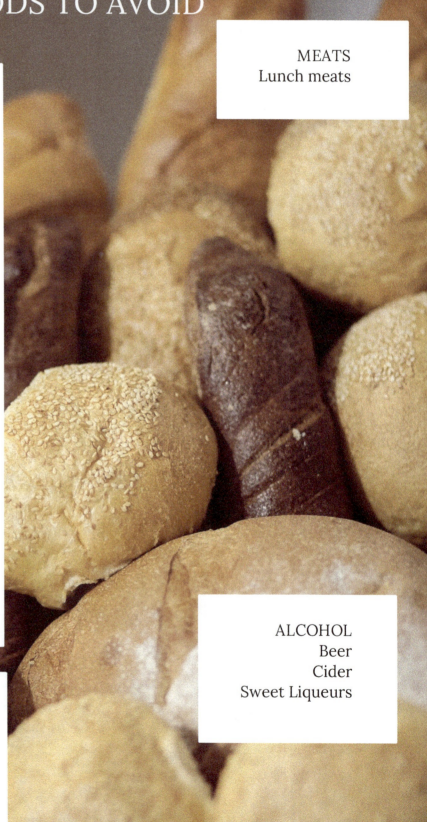

**GRAINS & STARCHES**
Barley
Bread
Breakfast cereals
Buckwheat
Bulgur wheat
Chickpeas
Corn
Couscous
Crackers
Dried beans
Lentils
Legumes
Millet
Muesli
Oats
Pasta
Peas
Pies
Pizza
Potatoes
Quinoa
Rice
Rye
Wheat Flour
Whole Wheat Flour

**MEATS**
Lunch meats

**ALCOHOL**
Beer
Cider
Sweet Liqueurs

**FATS**
Canola Oil
Cottonseed Oil
Corn Oil
Flaxseed Oil

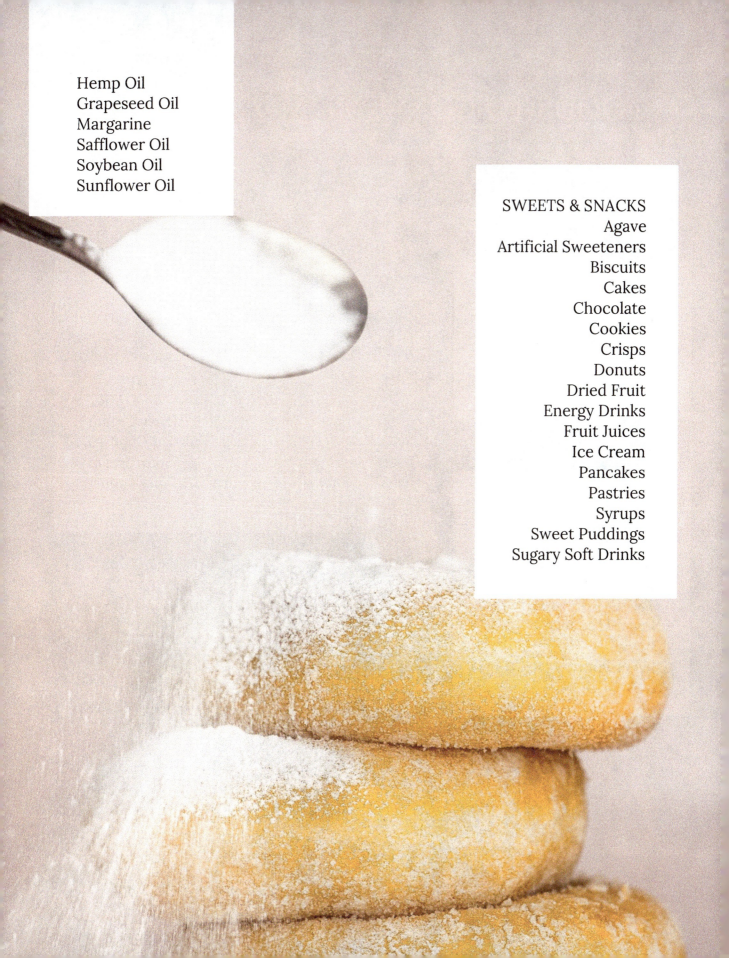

Hemp Oil
Grapeseed Oil
Margarine
Safflower Oil
Soybean Oil
Sunflower Oil

SWEETS & SNACKS
Agave
Artificial Sweeteners
Biscuits
Cakes
Chocolate
Cookies
Crisps
Donuts
Dried Fruit
Energy Drinks
Fruit Juices
Ice Cream
Pancakes
Pastries
Syrups
Sweet Puddings
Sugary Soft Drinks

# FOODS TO CONSUME MODERATELY

ALCOHOL
Brandy
Dry Red or White Wine
Gin
Tequila
Vodka
Whiskey

NUTS
Chestnuts
Cashew Nuts
Peanuts
Pistachios

DAIRY
Heavy Cream
Full-Fat Cheeses
Sour Cream
Unsweetened Greek & Plain Yogurt

FRUIT & SWEETENERS
All the other fruits
Dark Chocolate
Diet Sodas
Erythritol
Honey
Sugar-Free Jello
Stevia
Sweet Potato

# *Your Journey Starts Right Here*

We have seen how the ketogenic diet is a relatively safe and super effective way to lose weight and improve several symptoms. For women over 50, it has even more advantages. Investigations are still ongoing, and my commitment is to keep this book up to date with the latest information available.

In my 20+ years' experience, I have seen wonderful results with this protocol, and I hope you will put into practice all the theory (this is what the recipes, the meal plan, and journal are meant for!).

Women over 50 are a lot more sensitive to lifestyle changes due to fluctuating hormones. This means that you could already have experienced frustration while trying a diet and getting little to no results. It is important to realize that not everybody should approach the keto diet in the same way: some will experience a more or less intense "keto flu" at the beginning, others will just have a steady weight loss while still enjoying the food they love... for others will be difficult to stick to the diet after the first week.

The ketogenic diet is clinically proven to produce astounding results in those who follow its principles and are consistent with its application. At the end of the day, whether it will work or not depend on just one variable: You.

I decided to create some powerful tools to accompany you on this Journey: you have basically no excuse to start the ketogenic diet TODAY.

After this chapter, you will find 75 keto-friendly recipes, specifically adapted for the needs of women over 50.

Now it is time to leave the theory behind and get started with the practice!

.

# SCIENTIFIC REFERENCES

- Freeman JM, Kossoff EH, Hartman AL. The ketogenic diet: one decade later. Pediatrics. 2007
- Martin-McGill KJ, Jackson CF, Bresnahan R, Levy RG, Cooper PN. Ketogenic diets for drug-resistant epilepsy. Cochrane Database Syst Rev. 2018
- Gano LB, Patel M, Rho JM. Ketogenic diets, mitochondria, and neurological diseases. J Lipid Res. 2014
- Huttenlocher PR, Wilbourn AJ, Signore JM. Medium-chain triglycerides as a therapy for intractable childhood epilepsy. *Neurology*. 1971
- Neal EG, Chaffe H, Schwartz RH, Lawson MS, Edwards N, Fitzsimmons G, *et al*. The ketogenic diet for the treatment of childhood epilepsy: a randomised controlled trial. Lancet Neurol. 2008
- Vining EP, Freeman JM, Ballaban-Gil K, Camfield CS, Camfield PR, Holmes GL, *et al*. A multicenter study of the efficacy of the ketogenic diet. Arch Neurol. 1998
- Kossoff EH, Zupec-Kania BA, Rho JM. Ketogenic diets: an update for child neurologists. J Child Neurol. 2009
- Kossoff EH, Zupec-Kania BA, Auvin S, Ballaban-Gil KR, Christina Bergqvist AG, Blackford R, Buchhalter JR, Caraballo RH, Cross JH, Dahlin MG, Donner EJ, Guzel O, Jehle RS, Klepper J, Kang HC, Lambrechts DA, Liu YMC, Nathan JK, Nordli DR Jr, Pfeifer HH, Rho JM, Scheffer IE, Sharma S, Stafstrom CE, Thiele EA, Turner Z, Vaccarezza MM, van der Louw EJTM, Veggiotti P, Wheless JW, Wirrell EC; Charlie Foundation; Matthew's Friends; Practice Committee of the Child Neurology Society. Optimal clinical management of children receiving dietary therapies for epilepsy: Updated recommendations of the International Ketogenic Diet Study Group. Epilepsia Open. 2018
- Husari KS, Cervenka MC. The ketogenic diet all grown up-Ketogenic diet therapies for adults. Epilepsy Res. 2020
- Hartman AL, Vining EP. Clinical aspects of the ketogenic diet. Epilepsia. 2007
- Freeman JM, Vining EP, Pillas DJ, Pyzik PL, Casey JC, Kelly LM. The efficacy of the ketogenic diet–1998: a prospective evaluation of intervention in 150 children. Pediatrics. 1998
- Laffel, Lori (November 1999). "Ketone bodies: a review of physiology, pathophysiology and application of monitoring to diabetes". Diabetes/Metabolism Research and Reviews.
- Ward C (2015). "Ketone Body Metabolism". Diapedia. Archived from the original on 2018-11-11. Retrieved 30 September 2019.
- Mattson MP, Moehl K, Ghena N, Schmaedick M, Cheng A (2018). "Intermittent metabolic switching, neuroplasticity and brain health". Nature Reviews. Neuroscience
- Westman, Eric C.; Tondt, Justin; Maguire, Emily; Yancy, William S. (15 September 2018). "Implementing a low-carbohydrate, ketogenic diet to manage type 2 diabetes mellitus". Expert Review of Endocrinology & Metabolism
- Ketogenic diet improves metabolic syndrome in multiple ways, diabetes.co.uk, Dec. 2017
- Gershuni, Victoria M.; Yan, Stephanie L.; Medici, Valentina (20 August 2018). "Nutritional Ketosis for Weight Management and Reversal of Metabolic Syndrome". Current Nutrition Reports
- Krebs, H.A. (January 1966). "The regulation of the release of ketone bodies by the liver". Advances in Enzyme Regulation

- Cahill GF (2006). "Fuel metabolism in starvation". Annual Review of Nutrition.
- Paoli A, Rubini A, Volek JS, Grimaldi KA (2013). "Beyond weight loss: a review of the therapeutic uses of very-low-carbohydrate (ketogenic) diets". European Journal of Clinical Nutrition

# PART 2

# Keto Diet Recipes

Prep time

Servings

Please note that nutrition facts and prep time may vary when ingredients are indicated as "to taste" and/or according to the temperature or kitchen tool used.

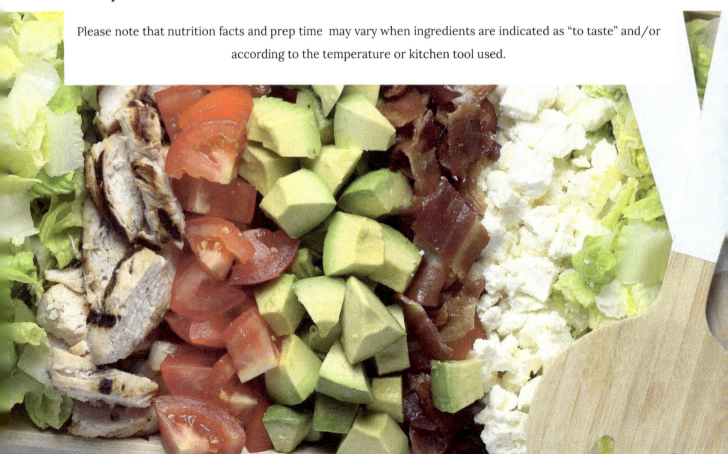

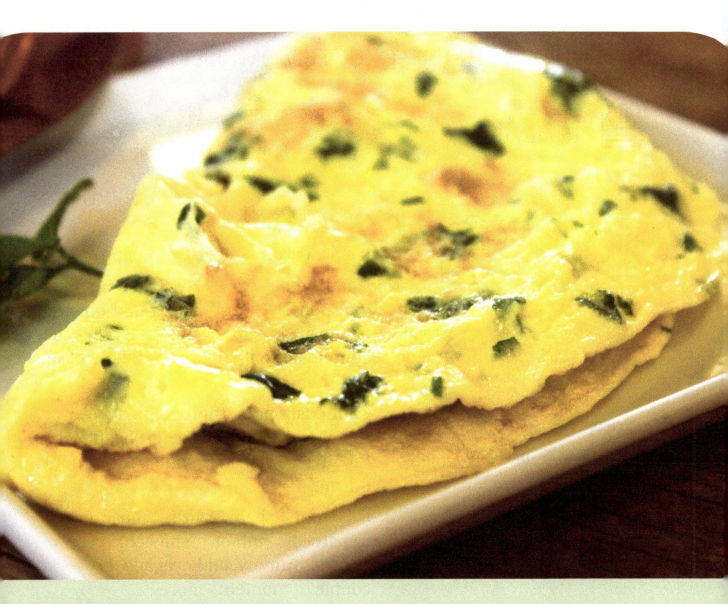

# BREAKFAST RECIPES

Breakfast

## JILL'S CHEESE-CRUSTED OMELETTE

 15 minutes

Calories per serving: 180

Carbs: 2g  Proteins: 13g  Fat: 41g

### INGREDIENTS

FOR THE OMELETTE

- 2 eggs
- 2 tbsp. (30 ml) heavy whipping cream
- salt and ground black pepper
- 1 tbsp. (15 ml) butter or coconut oil
- 3 oz. (75 g) (150 ml) mature shredded cheese or sliced

FOR THE FILLING

- 2 mushrooms, sliced
- 2 cherry tomatoes, sliced
- ½ oz. (15 g) (125 ml) baby spinach
- 2 tbsp. (30 ml) cream cheese
- 1 oz. (30 g) deli turkey

### DIRECTIONS

- Whisk together eggs and cream in a bowl. Season with salt and pepper.
- Heat the margarine over medium heat in a non-stick griddle. Spread out the cheddar in an even layer in the container, so it covers the whole base. Fry on medium heat until boiling.
- Cautiously pour the egg mixture over the cheddar and lower the heat. Cook for a couple of moments without mixing.
- Fill one half with mushrooms, tomatoes, infant spinach, cream cheddar, turkey, and oregano. Fry for a couple of moments more.
- At the point when the egg blend begins to set, turn the unfilled half over the garnish side, shaping a sickle. Fry for a couple of more minutes, and enjoy!

Breakfast

# CLASSIC BACON AND EGGS

 10 minutes     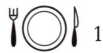 1

## INGREDIENTS

- 8 eggs
- 5 oz. (150 g) bacon, in slices
- cherry tomatoes (optional)
- fresh parsley (optional)

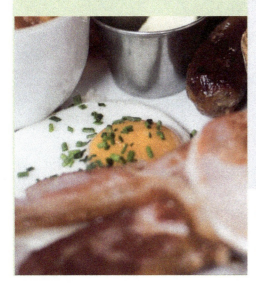

## DIRECTIONS

- Fry the bacon in a dish at medium-high temperature until fresh. Set aside on a plate. Leave the fat in the container.
- Use a similar skillet to sear the eggs. Place it at medium temperature and break your eggs into the bacon oil. You can likewise break them into an measuring cup and cautiously fill the container to try not to splatter hot oil.
- Cook the eggs any way you like them. You can leave the eggs to sear on one side and cover the dish to ensure they get cooked on top. Cut the cherry tomatoes down the middle and fry them at the same time.
- Salt and pepper to taste.

Calories per serving:     210

Carbs: 0g     Proteins: 15g     Fat: 16g

Breakfast

# SCRAMBLED EGGS

 5 minutes

## INGREDIENTS

- 1 oz. (30g) butter
- 2 eggs
- salt and pepper

 4

## DIRECTIONS

- Break the eggs into a little bowl and use a fork to whisk them along with some salt and pepper.
- Dissolve the butter in a non-stick skillet over medium temperature. Watch cautiously: the spread shouldn't turn brown!
- Pour the eggs into the skillet and mix for 1–2 minutes, until they are velvety.

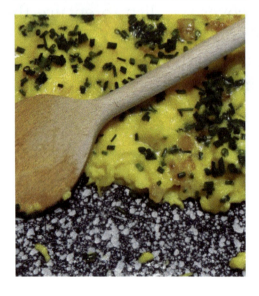

Calories per serving:   110

Carbs: 1g    Proteins: 15g    Fat: 4.5g

Breakfast

# EGG BUTTER WITH SMOKED SALMON AND AVOCADO

 20 minutes

## INGREDIENTS

- 4 eggs
- ½ tsp (2ml) sea salt
- ¼ tsp (1ml) ground black pepper
- 5 oz. (150 g) butter, at room temperature
- 2 avocados
- 2 tbsp. olive oil
- 1 tbsp. (4 g) fresh parsley, chopped
- 4 oz. (110 g) smoked salmon

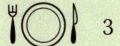 3

## DIRECTIONS

- Place the eggs in a pot cautiously. Cover with cold water and place on the oven without a lid. Heat the water to the point of boiling.
- Lower the heat and let stew for 7-8 minutes. Remove the eggs from the warm water and place them in a bowl with super cold water to cool.
- Strip the eggs and slash them finely. Blend eggs and margarine in with a fork. Season to taste with salt, pepper, or other seasonings of your choice.
- Serve the egg spread with a side of diced avocado, season with olive oil and finely hacked parsley, and smoked salmon.

Calories per serving:    190

Carbs: 4g    Proteins: 15g    Fat: 14g

Breakfast

# OMELET WRAP WITH SALMON & AVOCADO

30 minutes

Calories per serving: 280

Carbs: 5g    Proteins: 0g    Fat: 30g

## INGREDIENTS

- 3 large eggs
- 1/2 large avocado (100 g/ 3.5 oz.)
- 1/2 package smoked salmon (50 g/ 1.8 oz.)
- 2 heaped tbsp. full-fat cream cheese (64 g/ 2.3 oz.)
- 2 tbsp. (30ml) freshly chopped chives
- 1 medium spring onion, chopped (15 g/ 0.5 oz.)
- 1 tbsp. (15ml) ghee or butter
- sea salt & pepper, to taste

## DIRECTIONS

- Break the eggs into a blending bowl with a touch of salt and pepper and beat them well with a whisk or fork.
- Blend the cream cheese with chopped chives. Cut the smoked salmon and the avocado.
- Pour the eggs equally in a hot skillet lubed with ghee or butter. Cook at medium-low temperature. Try not to cook it quickly, or the omelet will be excessively dry.
- Use a spatula to take the egg from the sides towards the centre for the first 30 seconds. Cook. Make sure you don't cook the omelet for too long. The ideal surface ought to be delicate, and softened.
- Slide the omelet onto a plate and spoon the cream cheese.
- Add the salmon, avocado, chopped spring onion and overlap into a wrap.
- Serve right away or store in the fridge for as long as 1 day.

Breakfast

# SULLIVAN'S DOUGH BREAKFAST PIZZA

Calories per serving: 302

Carbs: 5g  Proteins: 15.7g  Fat: 26.1g

**FOR THE CRUST**
- ½ cup (125 ml) whey isolate unflavored protein powder (50 g)
- ½ tsp (2.5 g) baking powder
- ½ tsp (2 ml) granulated garlic
- ½ tsp (2 ml) salt
- ½ tsp (2 ml) Italian seasoning (blend of basil, oregano, rosemary, thyme, garlic powder, sage, coriander)
- 3 oz. (75 g) (125 ml) grated parmesan cheese
- 3 oz. (75 g) (150 ml) mozzarella cheese
- 2 oz. (50g) cream cheese
- 4 tbsp. olive oil
- 1 egg

**FOR THE TOPPING**
- 4 oz. (110 g) cream cheese
- 4 tbsp. (2 oz./ 60 ml) unsweetened tomato sauce
- 2 eggs scrambled
- 8 oz. (225 g) fresh sausage
- 3 oz. (75 g) chopped bacon
- 8 oz. (225 g) (475 ml) shredded cheddar cheese

1    25 minutes

## DIRECTIONS

- Preheat oven to 375°F (190°C).
- Mix all the ingredients for the crust in a large bowl until you get a thick batter.
- Use a wooden spoon or spatula to smooth the batter into a 9" round pizza.
- Heat the crust for 9 to 12 minutes until it turns golden brown.
- Remove the crust from the oven, and top with the indicated ingredients.
- Once done, bake again for 10-15 minutes, or until the toppings are seared and the cheddar is completely melted.

Breakfast

# PANCAKES WITH BERRIES AND WHIPPED CREAM

 25 minutes    4

Calories per serving: 160

Carbs: 10g   Proteins: 9g   Fat: 11g

### INGREDIENTS
**FOR THE PANCAKES**

- 4 eggs
- 7 oz. (200 g) (225 ml) cottage cheese
- 1 tbsp. (10 g) ground psyllium husk powder
- 2 oz. (50 g) butter or coconut oil

**FOR THE TOPPING**

- 2 oz. (50 g) fresh raspberries or blueberries or strawberries
- 1 cup (225 ml) heavy whipping cream

### DIRECTIONS

- Add eggs, cheese, and psyllium husk powder to a medium-size bowl and mix. Let sit for 5-10 minutes.
- Heat up butter or coconut oil in a non-stick skillet. Fry the pancakes on medium-low temperature for 3-4 minutes on each side. Try not to make them too big, or it will be difficult to flip them.
- Add the heavy whipping cream to a different bowl and whip until delicate pinnacles form.
- Serve the pancakes with your preferred whipped cream and berries!

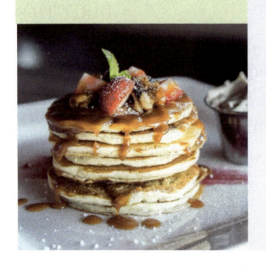

Breakfast

# FRITTATA WITH FRESH SPINACH

45 minutes

4

### INGREDIENTS

- 5 oz. (150 g) diced bacon or chorizo
- 2 tbsp. butter
- 8 oz. (225 g) (1.75 liters) fresh spinach
- 8 eggs
- 1 cup (225 ml) heavy whipping cream
- 5 oz. (150 g) (325 ml) shredded cheese
- salt and pepper

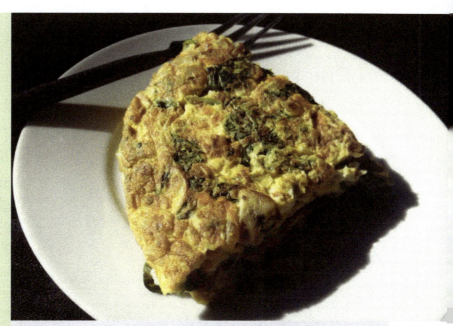

Calories per serving: 661

Carbs: 4g

Proteins: 27g

Fat: 59g

### DIRECTIONS

- Preheat oven to 350°F (175°C). Oil a 9x9 baking dish.
- Fry the bacon over medium heat until fresh. Add the spinach and mix. Then, remove from the oven.
- Whisk the eggs and cream together and fill the baking dish.
- Add the bacon, spinach, and cheddar on top and place in the oven once again. Cook for 25–30 minutes.
- Serve!

Breakfast

# MUSHROOM AND CHEESE FRITTATA

45 minutes

4

Calories per serving: 80

Carbs: 6g   Proteins: 4g   Fat: 4g

## INGREDIENTS

### FOR THE FRITTATA

- 1 lb. (450 g) mushrooms
- 4 oz. (110 g) butter
- 6 scallions
- 1 tbsp. (4 g) fresh parsley
- 1 tsp salt
- ½ tsp ground black pepper
- 10 eggs
- 8 oz. (225 g) (475 ml) shredded cheese
- 1 cup (225g) mayonnaise
- 4 oz. (110 g) (475 ml) leafy greens

### FOR THE VINAIGRETTE

- 4 tbsp. (60 ml) olive oil
- 1 tbsp. (15 ml) white wine vinegar
- ½ tsp (2 ml) salt
- ¼ tsp (1 ml) ground black pepper

## DIRECTIONS

- Preheat oven to 350°F (175°C).
- Set aside the vinaigrette ingredients in a bowl.
- Cut the mushrooms as you prefer.
- Sauté the mushrooms on medium-high temperature. Lower the heat. Save some butter to lube the baking dish.
- Take the scallions and mix with the seared mushrooms. Add salt and pepper to taste, and blend in the parsley.
- Blend eggs, mayonnaise, and cheddar in a different bowl. Add salt and pepper to taste.
- Add the mushrooms and scallions and put everything into a round, lubed baking dish. Cook for 30–40 minutes until the frittata turns bright yellow.
- Let cool for 5 minutes and serve with leafy greens and vinaigrette.

Breakfast

# ALL DAY KETO BREAKFAST

25 minutes

## INGREDIENTS

- 1 large egg
- 4 to 5 thin-cut (60 g/ 2.1 oz.) or 2 regular slices bacon
- 4 to 5 brown mushrooms (84 g/ 3 oz.) or 1 large Portobello mushroom
- 1/2 (100 g/ 3.5 oz.) large avocado
- 1 tbsp. (15 ml) ghee or duck fat
- salt and pepper, to taste

## DIRECTIONS

- Heat a skillet lubed with ghee over medium-high temperature. Cook the mushrooms for around 5 minutes. Flip and cook for around 2 more minutes. Move to a plate.
- Fry the bacon. Then, fry the egg until the white is cooked, and the yolk is as yet runny.
- Add avocado.
- Season to taste and serve right away!

Calories per serving: 580

Carbs: 11g    Proteins: 25g    Fat: 50g

Breakfast

# BREAKFAST SANDWICH

25 minutes

Calories per serving: 730

Carbs: 16g   Proteins: 45g   Fat: 58g

## INGREDIENTS

- 2 sausage patties
- 1 egg
- 1 tbsp. (15 ml) cream cheese
- 2 tbsp. (30 ml) sharp cheddar
- 1/4 (1 ml) medium avocado, sliced
- 1/4–1/2 tsp (2 ml) sriracha (to taste)
- Salt, pepper to taste

## DIRECTIONS

- In a skillet over medium temperature, cook the patties following the label directions and set aside.
- In a little bowl, add cream cheese and sharp cheddar. Microwave for 20-30 seconds until melted.
- Mix cheddar with sriracha and set aside.
- With the egg, make a little omelet.
- Fill omelet with cheddar + sriracha blend and serve as a sandwich.

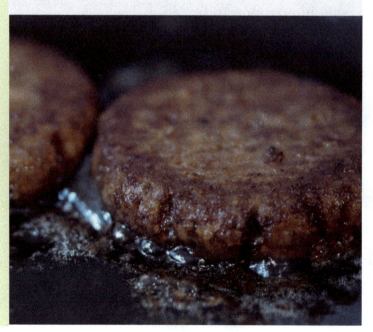

Breakfast

# KETO CORNBREAD

35 minutes

## INGREDIENTS

- 1/2 cup (75 g) almond flour
- 1/4 cup (35 g) coconut flour
- 1 tsp (5 ml) salt
- 1/2 tsp (2.5 ml) baking soda
- 3 large eggs
- 1/2 cup (120 ml) (4 oz.) heavy cream
- 1/4 cup (60 ml) (2 oz.) butter melted
- Optional Fillings
- 2 jalapeños thinly sliced
- 4 slices bacon cooked and crumbled
- 1/2 cup (125ml) shredded cheddar cheese

- Preheat oven to 325°F (170°C).
- Mix all the ingredients together in a medium bowl except the jalapeños.
- In a 10.5″ cast-iron skillet, pour the batter and add jalapeños; bake for 25-30 minutes. Before cutting and serving, let cool for 5 minutes.

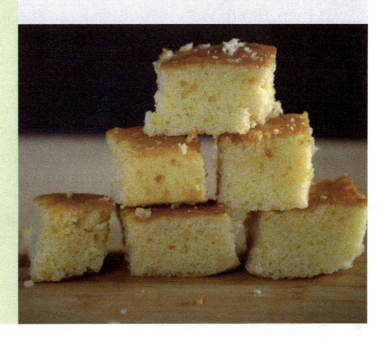

Calories per serving:     110

Carbs: 8g     Proteins: 4g     Fat: 6g

Breakfast

# TOMATO BAKED EGGS

60 minutes          4

## INGREDIENTS

- 3.6 cup (900 g) vine-ripened tomatoes
- 3 garlic cloves
- 3 tbsp. (50 ml) olive oil
- 4 large free-range eggs
- 2 tbsp. (30 ml) chopped parsley and/or chives

## DIRECTIONS

- Preheat oven to 360°F/390°F (180°C/200°C). Cut the tomatoes into quarters and put them into a baking dish. Sprinkle over the cut garlic.
- Sprinkle with the olive oil, season well with salt and pepper, and mix everything together.
- Put the dish into the oven and cook for 40 minutes until the tomatoes get bright colored.
- Carve four holes in the mixture, break an egg into each hole, and cover the dish with a sheet of foil.
- Put it back to the oven for 5-10 minutes until the eggs are set. Sprinkle over the spices and serve hot. You can accompany it with warm crusty bread and a serving of mixed greens.

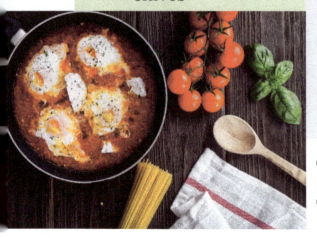

Calories per serving:     184

Carbs: 11g     Proteins: 15g     Fat: 10g

Breakfast

# CHOCOLATE PANCAKE CEREAL

Calories per serving: 160

25 minutes  4

Carbs: 10g   Proteins: 9g   Fat: 11g

## INGREDIENTS

- 1/4 cup coconut flour (30 g/ 1.1 oz.)
- 1/2 cup cacao powder or Dutch process cocoa powder (43 g/ 1.5 oz.)
- 1/2 tsp gluten-free baking powder
- Optional: 2-4 tbsp. granulated Erythritol
- 1/4 cup unsweetened coconut yogurt or full-fat yogurt (60 ml/ 2 fl oz.)
- 3 tbsp. melted virgin coconut oil, divided (45 ml)
- 4 large eggs
- Optional: chopped dark chocolate, sugar-free maple-flavored syrup, berries, butter, almond butter, whipped cream, almond milk, or Keto Condensed Milk to serve

## DIRECTIONS

- Place all the dry ingredients into a large blending bowl and mix to combine and remove any knots.
- Combine the yogurt with 1 tbsp. (15 ml) coconut oil and eggs in another bowl; then mix with the dry ingredients.
- Blend well until the batter is smooth.
- Heat a skillet over medium-high temperature and oil with a tsp of the excess coconut oil, or use coconut oil dip. (more oil is needed for a cast iron skillet; less for a non-stick skillet).
- Make little spheres, approx. 2 cm (3/4"). Cook them for just about 1 minute, then flip.
- Serve with your favorite dressings: chopped dim chocolate, almond butter, yogurt, or Keto Condensed Milk.

*Store, in a closed container, in the fridge for as long as 5 days*

Breakfast

# EASY BANANA MUFFINS

## INGREDIENTS

- 250 g (1 cup) self-rising flour
- 1 tsp (5 ml) baking powder
- ½ tsp (2 ml) bicarbonate of soda
- 110 g (2/3 cup or 4 oz.) caster sugar
- 75 g (1/3 cup) butter, melted
- 1 tsp (5 ml) vanilla extract
- 2 eggs
- 2 large ripe bananas, mashed
- 125 ml (½ cup) buttermilk (or add 1 tsp lemon juice to milk and leave for 20 min)
- 50 g (1/3 cup) pecans, chopped, plus extra to decorate (optional)

## DIRECTIONS

- Preheat oven to 350°F (175°C).
- Grease a muffin tin.
- Sift flour, baking powder, bicarbonate of soda, and caster sugar with a touch of salt.
- In a different bowl, blend the melted butter, vanilla extract, eggs, bananas, and buttermilk.
- Mix together dry and wet ingredients.
- Top with pecans.
- Heat for 20-25 min, until golden brown.
- Let cool and serve.

Calories per serving: 170

Carbs: 27g

Proteins: 3g

Fat: 6g

25 mins    12

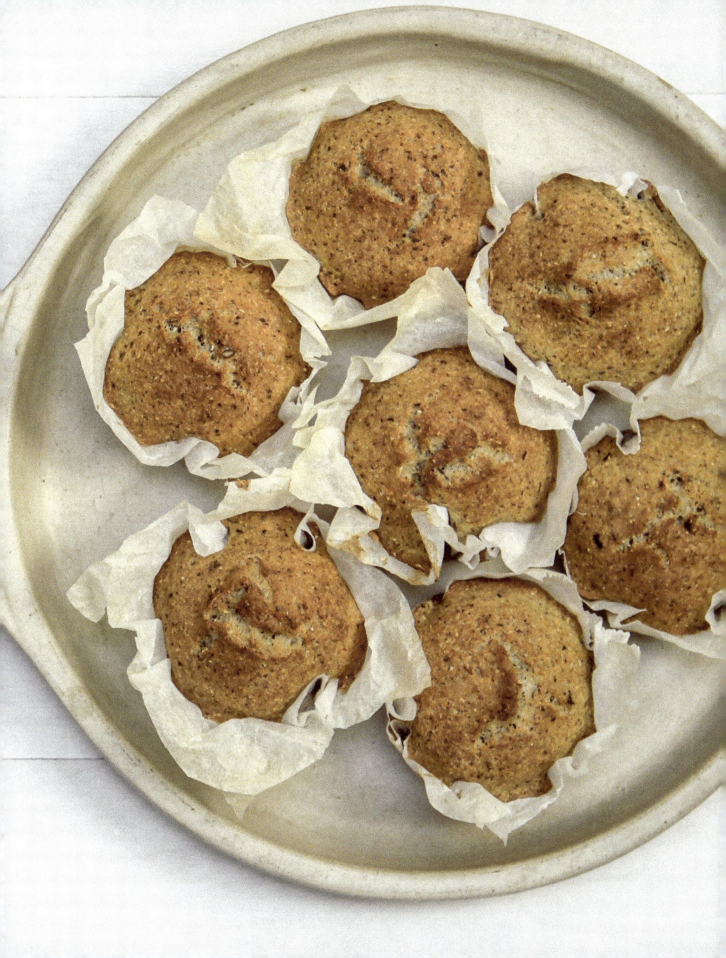

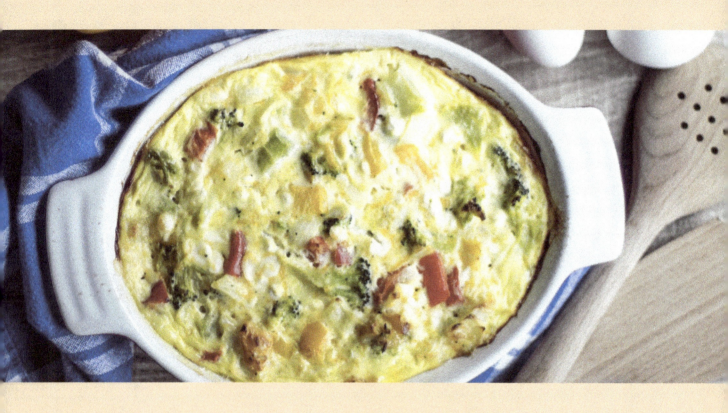

# MAIN MEALS

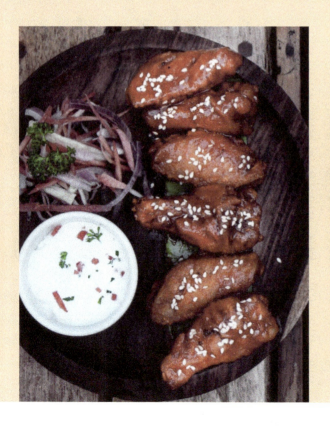
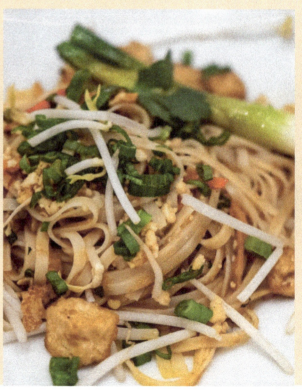

Main meals

# CHICKEN CURRY PIE

70 mins

4

## INGREDIENTS

**PIE CRUST**

- ¾ cup (175 ml) (75 g) almond flour
- 4 tbsp. (35g) sesame seeds
- 4 tbsp. (25ml) coconut flour
- 1 tbsp. (10 g) psyllium husk powder
- 1 tsp (5 ml) baking powder
- 1 p" salt
- 3 tbsp. (50 ml) olive oil or coconut oil
- 1 egg
- 4 tbsp. water

**FILLING**

- 11 oz. (300 g) cooked chicken
- 1 cup (225 ml) mayonnaise
- 3 eggs
- ½ (70 g) green bell pepper chopped
- 1 tbsp. curry powder
- 1 tsp (5 ml) paprika powder
- 1 tsp (1 ml) onion powder
- ¼ tsp (1 ml) ground black pepper
- 4 oz. (110 g) cream cheese
- 1¼ cup (300 ml) (150 g) shredded cheese

## DIRECTIONS

- Preheat oven to 350°F (175°C). Put all the ingredients for the pie into a food processor for a couple of moments until the mixture solidifies into a ball. If you don't have a food processor, you can likewise blend the mixture with a fork or by hand.

- Lay out some baking paper onto a spring-form pan, no bigger than 10" (23 cm) (the spring-form pan makes it simpler to remove the pie when it's ready). Oil base and sides of the container.

- Spread the batter into the container. Use an oiled spatula or your fingers. Pre-heat the outside layer for 10–15 minutes.

- Mix all the other ingredients together, and fill the outside layer. Cook for 35–40 minutes.

- Let it cool 20 minutes before serving.

Calories per serving: 330

Carbs: 12g    Proteins: 35g    Fat: 16g

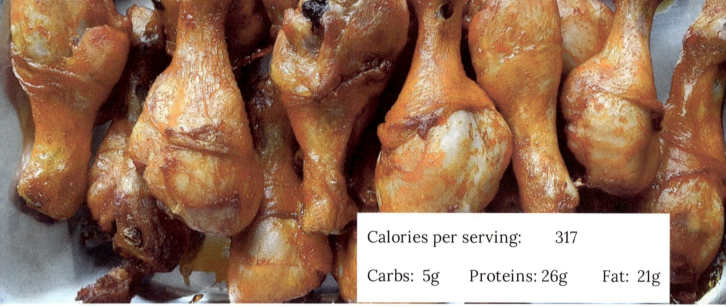

Calories per serving: 317

Carbs: 5g   Proteins: 26g   Fat: 21g

# BUFFALO DRUMSTICKS WITH CHILI AIOLI

 50 mins

 4

## CHICKEN DRUMSTICKS AND MARINADE

- 2 lb. (900 g) chicken drumsticks
- 2 tbsp. (30 ml) olive oil or coconut oil
- 2 tbsp. (30 ml) white wine vinegar
- 1 tbsp. (15 ml) tomato paste
- 1 tsp (5 ml) salt
- 1 tsp (5 ml) paprika powder
- 1 tbsp. (15 ml) tabasco

## CHILI AIOLI

- 1/3 cup (75 ml) mayonnaise
- 2 tsp (10 ml) chipotle powder
- 1 garlic clove, minced

## DIRECTIONS

### Chicken drumsticks and marinade

- Preheat oven to 365°F (185°C). Oil a cooking dish.
- Put the drumsticks in a medium-sized bowl.
- Mix the marinade fixings together in a little bowl, and afterward, pour it over the wings to totally cover. Marinade for 10 minutes at room temperature.
- Place the drumsticks in the baking dish and cook for 30-40 minutes, until golden and fresh.

### Chili aioli

- In a little bowl, combine the mayonnaise, minced garlic, and stew powder until combined.
- Serve the wings with the aioli.

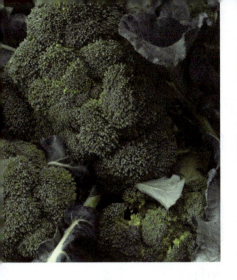
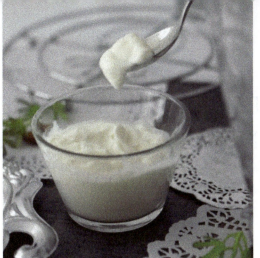
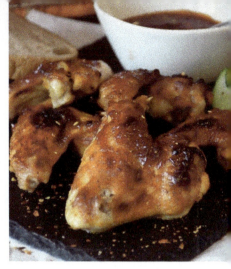

## CHICKEN WINGS WITH CREAMY BROCCOLI

55 mins

4

### DIRECTIONS

- Baked chicken wings
- ½ (70 g) orange, juice and zest
- ¼ cup (60 ml) olive oil
- 2 tsp (30 ml) ground ginger
- 1 tsp (5 ml) salt
- ¼ tsp cayenne pepper
- 3 lb. (1440 g) chicken wings
- Creamy broccoli
- 1½ lb. (650 g) broccoli
- 1 cup (225 ml) mayonnaise
- ¼ cup (60 ml) (2.25 g) chopped fresh dill
- salt and pepper, to taste

- Preheat oven to 400°F (200°C).
- Mix orange juice and zest with oil in a little bowl. Place the chicken wings in a plastic box and pour in the marinade.
- Shake the box so as to cover the wings completely. Set aside to marinate for 5 minutes or more, if needed.
- Place the wings in a single layer in a lubed cooking dish.
- Bake for around 45 minutes until the wings take on a bright color.
- In the meanwhile, parboil the broccoli in salted water for a few minutes. They're simply supposed to soften a little bit but not lose their shape or shading.
- Drain the broccoli and let cool before adding the extra ingredients. Serve the broccoli with the cooked wings.

Calories per serving:    660

Carbs: 3g   Proteins: 31g    Fat: 53g

Main meals

# PEPPER-CRUSTED BEEF TENDERLOIN WITH HERBED STEAK SAUCE

65 mins    4

## INGREDIENTS

**BEEF**

- 2 lb. (900 g) beef, tenderloin
- 2 tsp (10 ml) garlic powder
- 2 tsp (10 ml) onion powder
- 1 tbsp. (15 ml) black peppercorns, coarsely ground
- ½ tsp (2 ml) salt
- 2 tbsp. (30 ml) olive oil

**SAUCE**

- 9 oz. (250 g) butter
- 1 tbsp. (15 ml) lemon juice
- 1 tsp (5 ml) garlic cloves, minced
- 2 tbsp. (8 g) fresh parsley, chopped
- 1 tbsp. (15 ml) Dijon mustard
- 1 tsp (5 ml) smoked paprika powder
- 1 tsp (5 ml) dried thyme
- 1 tsp (5 ml) dried oregano
- 1 tbsp. fresh chives, finely chopped
- salt and pepper to taste

## DIRECTIONS

**MEAT**

- Mix the meat dressings together in a little bowl.
- Sprinkle the mixture on a foil and roll the hamburgers on it until they are completely covered.
- Set aside and let rest for 30 minutes.
- Heat skillet gril or BBQ over medium-high temperature.
- Drizzle the meat with olive oil and burn on each side for approx. 5-7 minutes.
- Allow meat to rest for 15 minutes before cutting.

**SAUCE**

- Over medium-low temperature, add all the sauce ingredients into a little pot and mix delicately until the spread melts.
- Whisk well, add to the meat and serve with a green plate of mixed greens or steamed vegetables.

Calories per serving: 300

Carbs: 4g    Proteins: 47g    Fat: 17g

Main meals

# MEXICAN CAULIFLOWER RICE

### INGREDIENTS

- 3 oz. (85 g) Butter
- 1 1/2 tsp garlic powder
- 3 tsp onion flakes
- 1/2 tsp pepper
- 1/2 tsp salt
- 2 cup (320 g) cauliflower rice
- 1/4 cup (65 g) tomato puree
- 2 tsp cilantro finely chopped

30 mins         4

### DIRECTIONS

- Place a large skillet over medium-low heat. Add margarine, garlic powder, and onion and delicately sauté for 3 minutes.
- Add the cauliflower rice, salt, and pepper and sauté for 3 minutes.
- Add the tomato puree and mix well. Keep on cooking for 3-5 minutes.
- Take the skillet off the heat and pour in the cilantro.
- Serve.

Calories per serving:     60

Carbs: 10g    Proteins: 3g    Fat: 2g

Main meals

# TACO PIE

40 mins

6

## INGREDIENTS

- 1.5 lb. (680.39 g) ground beef or turkey
- 1 egg
- 2 tbsp. taco seasoning
- 2 tbsp. coconut flour
- Toppings
- 8 oz. (226.8 g) shredded cheddar cheese divided
- 1 cup (260g) salsa
- 2 cup (144 g) chopped lettuce
- 1 cup (149 g) chopped tomato
- ⅓ cup (53.33 g) chopped onion
- ½ cup (118 g) Mexican cream or sour cream thinned with 1 tbsp. of almond milk

## DIRECTIONS

- Preheat oven to 400°F (200°C).
- Mix the ground meat with taco seasoning, coconut flour, and egg.
- Grease a baking dish. Top with half of the shredded cheddar.
- Cook for 25-30 minutes.
- Remove from the oven. Pour over the salsa and the remaining cheedar.
- Top with lettuce, tomato, and onion.
- Sprinkle on the cream and serve.

Calories per serving:     389

Carbs: 1g     Proteins: 20g     Fat: 32g

Main meals

# POT BARBECUE CHICKEN

## INGREDIENTS

- 4 lb. (1.81 kg) boneless skinless chicken thighs
- 1 tbsp. garlic powder
- 1 tbsp. onion powder
- 1 tbsp. smoked paprika
- 1 tsp salt
- ½ tsp pepper
- Sugar-free BBQ sauce for serving

## DIRECTIONS

- Add all the ingredients to the pot and blend well.
- Cook over high heat for 10 minutes.
- Move to a plate and let cool.
- Add BBQ sauce (optional) and serve.

Calories per serving: 519

Carbs: 0g

Proteins: 43g

Fat: 5g

20 mins

8

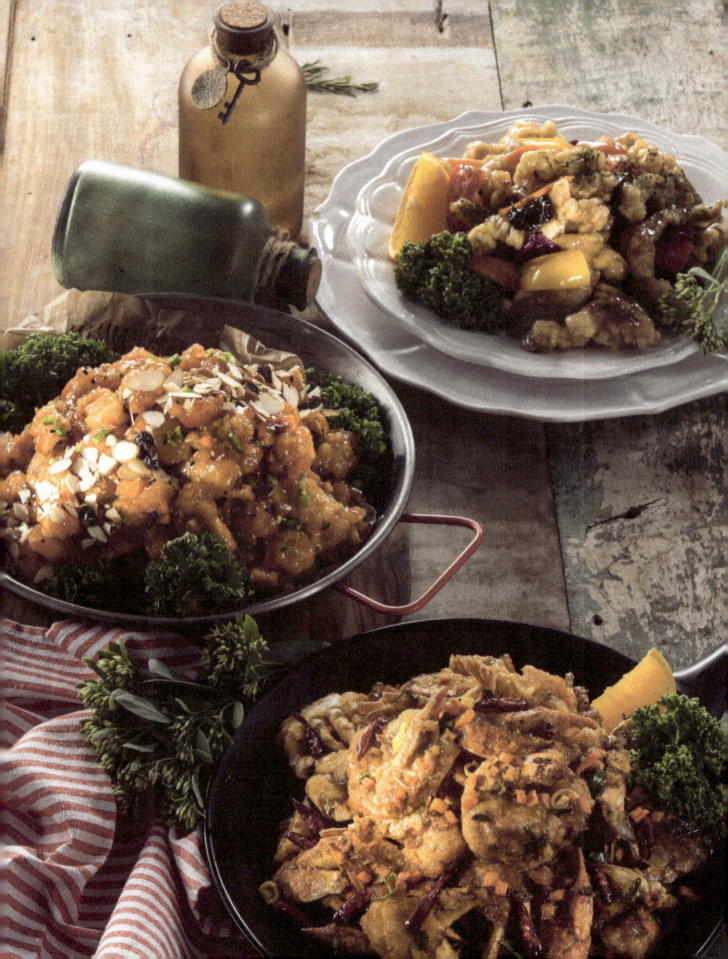

Main meals

# SPAGHETTI SQUASH CASSEROLE

35 mins

6

## INGREDIENTS

- 2 cup (143.42 g) cooked spaghetti squash
- 1 egg
- 1 tsp (4.93 g) herbs de provence (or a few p"es of thyme, rosemary and tarragon)
- 8 oz. onion and chive flavored cream cheese (or similar)
- p" of salt
- 1 cup (112g) mozzarella cheese

## DIRECTIONS

- Preheat oven to 350°F (180°C).
- Spray a baking dish with cooking spray.
- Put the cooked spaghetti squash in the dish.
- Combine the eggs, cream cheddar, spices, and salt in a blender. Mix until smooth. Pour over the spaghetti squash.
- Sprinkle the cheddar on top.
- Bake for 30-40 minutes.
- Let cool for 10 minutes and serve.

Calories per serving: 193

Carbs: 8g   Proteins: 20g   Fat: 10g

Main meals

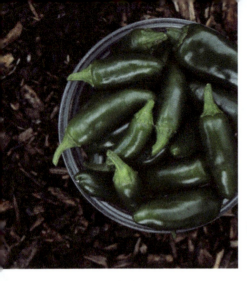

# JALAPENO POPPER CHICKEN CASSEROLE

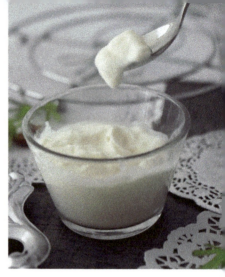

## INGREDIENTS

 45 mins     8

### CASSEROLE

- 2 lb. (907.18 g) chicken breasts cooked and chopped
- 8 oz. (226.8 g) cream cheese
- ½ cup (112 g) mayo
- ½ cup (115 g) sour cream
- ½ cup (56.5 g) shredded cheddar
- ½ cup (118.29 g) bacon crumbles
- ½ cup (74.5 g) jalapeno or poblano pepper seeded and diced
- 1 tsp garlic powder
- ½ tsp salt

### TOPPING

- ¼ cup (28.25 g) shredded cheddar
- ¼ cup (28.25 g) crumbled bacon
- 1 thinly sliced and seeded jalapeno (optional)

## DIRECTIONS

- Mix the casserole ingredients (except the chicken) in a large bowl.
- Blend until smooth. Put over cooked chicken.
- Put into an oiled baking dish. Top with cheddar, bacon, and cut jalapenos.
- Cook at 350°F (180°C) for 35 minutes until boiling.
- Serve with a portion of mixed greens.

Calories per serving:    553

Carbs: 4g     Proteins: 49g     Fat: 37g

Main meals

# KETO STIR FRY

30 mins      8

- 1 tbsp. oil
- 3 lb. (1.36 kg) chicken thighs cut into strips
- 1 zucchini sliced
- 1 yellow squash sliced
- 1 pepper sliced
- 1 onion sliced
- 12 oz. (340.2 g) green beans or 6 cup of any vegetables
- Teriyaki Sauce
- ¾ cup (180 g) soy sauce or coconut aminos
- ¼ cup (50 g) brown sugar substitute such as Golden Lakanto
- 1 tbsp. garlic chopped
- 1 tbsp. fresh ginger peeled and finely chopped
- 1 tbsp. apple cider vinegar
- To serve (optional)
- 16 oz. (453.59 g) cauliflower rice

## DIRECTIONS

- Heat oil in a large skillet over medium-high temperature. Add the onions and peppers.
- Add the zucchini, squash, and green beans. Cook until very soft.
- Move to a large serving bowl.
- Add the chicken to the skillet and sauté until completely cooked.
- Drain the cooking fluid.
- Add the vegetables to the skillet.
- Add the teriyaki sauce. Blend well.
- Serve with cauliflower rice.
- Note: to make Teriyaki Sauce, simply stir together all the ingredients.

Calories per serving: 262

Carbs: 9g    Proteins: 28g    Fat: 12g

Main meals

# CRISPY LEMON BAKED CHICKEN THIGHS

3hrs 50 mins

4

## INGREDIENTS

- 2 lb. (900 g) chicken thighs (bone-in with skin)
- 4 tbsp. (60 ml) olive oil
- 4 tbsp. (60 ml) lemon juice
- 2 tbsp. (30 ml) red wine vinegar
- 3 tbsp. (50 ml) fresh oregano, finely chopped
- 2 garlic cloves, minced
- 2 tsp salt
- ½ tsp (2 ml) ground black pepper
- 2 tsp fresh thyme, finely chopped

## DIRECTIONS

- Mix the marinade ingredients in a blending bowl. Add on the chicken thighs until completely covered.
- Place in the fridge for at least 3 hours.
- Preheat oven to 400°F/200°C.
- Remove the chicken thighs from the marinade, and put them skin-side up on the tray(s).
- Cook for 30-35 minutes, until the inside temperature is 165°F/74°C, and the skin is bright pink.
- Let rest for 5-10 minutes before serving.

Calories per serving: 270

Carbs: 0g   Proteins: 27g   Fat: 17g

Main meals

# PESTO CHICKEN CASSEROLE WITH FETA CHEESE AND OLIVES

## INGREDIENTS

- 1 ½ lb. (650 g) boneless chicken thighs
- salt and pepper
- 2 tbsp. butter or coconut oil
- 1/3 cup (70 ml) red pesto or green pesto
- 1¼ cup (300 ml) heavy whipping cream
- 3 oz. (75 g) (125 ml) pitted olives
- 5 oz. (150 g) feta cheese, diced
- 1 garlic clove, finely chopped
- For serving
- 5 oz. (150 g) (650 ml) leafy greens
- ¼ cup (60ml) olive oil
- sea salt and ground black pepper

## DIRECTIONS

- Preheat oven to 400°F (200°C).
- Cut the chicken into scaled-down pieces. Season with salt and pepper.
- Add margarine or oil to a large skillet and fry the chicken pieces at medium-high temperature.
- Mix pesto and heavy cream in a bowl.
- Place the seared chicken pieces in a cooking dish along with olives, feta cheddar, and garlic. Add the pesto/cream mixture.
- Bake in the oven for 20-30 minutes.

45 mins

4

Calories per serving: 300

Carbs: 11g   Proteins: 28g   Fat: 18g

Main meals

# STUFFED CHICKEN BREAST WITH ZOODLES AND TOMATO SAUCE

## DIRECTIONS

- Preheat oven to 400°F (200°C).
- Sauté the baby spinach until it shrinks.
- Add salt and pepper. Place in a bowl and blend in with the goat cheese.
- Slice the chicken breasts lengthwise. Place them on a lubed baking dish.
- Fill the chicken breasts with the ricotta cheese mixture and sprinkle the shredded cheddar on top. Add bits of the remaining butter.
- Bake in the oven for around 20–30 minutes, until the chicken turns golden brown.
- Fry shallot and onion in butter until soft. Add tomato paste, vinegar, crushed tomatoes, and bring to a boil. Add the spices. Let rest at low temperature for 15 minutes, then add salt and pepper to taste.
- Use a spiralizer to cut the zucchini or, if you don't have one, make thin zucchini strips with a potato peeler.
- Blend the zucchini in the tomatoes and serve with the chicken.

 60 mins     2

## STUFFED CHICKEN BREASTS

- 5 oz. (150 g) (1.2 l) baby spinach
- salt and pepper
- 8 oz. (225 g) goat cheese or ricotta cheese
- 4 chicken breasts (skinless)
- 1 cup (225 ml) (100 g) cheddar cheese, shredded
- 2 oz. (50 g) butter
- grated parmesan cheese

## TOMATO SAUCE

- 1 shallot, finely chopped
- 2 garlic cloves, minced
- 2 oz. (50 g) butter
- 2 tbsp. tomato paste
- ½ tbsp. (2 ml) red wine vinegar
- 14 oz. (475 ml) (475 g) crushed tomatoes
- 1 tsp dried basil
- 1 tsp dried oregano
- ½ tsp salt
- pepper, to taste
- 2 zucchinis (400 g) spiralized

Calories per serving:    206

Carbs: 0g

Proteins: 32g

Fat: 8g

Main meals

# CREAMY CHICKEN, BACON AND CAULIFLOWER BAKE

1 hr 5 mins

4

## INGREDIENTS

- 2 wooden skewers
- 10 oz. (100 g) Salami sliced thin
- 1/3 cup (80 g) Franks Hot Sauce

Calories per serving: 300

Carbs: 6g

Proteins: 34g

Fat: 34g

## DIRECTIONS

- Preheat oven to 400°F (200°C).
- Oil a large baking dish.
- Heat the olive oil and butter in a large skillet over medium until the butter is bubbling.
- Add the cauliflower and bacon. Cook, mixing occasionally, for 8-10 minutes.
- Add the spinach to the skillet. Cook, mixing, for other 2 minutes.
- Remove from heat and add cream, thyme, and half shallot. Then, move to a plate.
- Add the chicken to the skillet and cook for 2 minutes on each side until golden brown.
- Place on top of the cauliflower mixture.
- Sprinkle cheese over the chicken. Heat for 20-25 minutes.
- Serve with the remaining shallot.

Main meals

# CAULIFLOWER MASH

## INGREDIENTS

- 1 large cauliflower, trimmed, cut in florets
- 2 garlic cloves, peeled, smashed
- 1 tbsp. (15ml) olive oil
- 1/8 cup (200g) streaky bacon, coarsely chopped
- 1/3 cup (85g) sour cream
- 1 cup (80g) coarsely grated cheddar
- 1 tbsp. chopped fresh chives, plus extra to sprinkle
- Melted butter, to serve

## DIRECTIONS

- Bring a large pot of water to a boil.
- Add the cauliflower and garlic and cook for 10-15 minutes.
- Then, heat the oil in a skillet over medium heat. Add the bacon and cook for 4 minutes. Set aside.
- Preheat oven to 360°F (180°C). Put the cauliflower mixture in a food processor until fine pieces form. Move to a medium bowl. Mix through the sour cream, a large portion of the cheddar, and chives.
- Place the cauliflower mixture in a round 20cm baking dish. Top with the remaining cheddar and the bacon.
- Cook for 10 minutes until the cheddar is melted.
- Sprinkle with additional chives. Top with melted butter.

20 mins            4

Calories per serving:     199

Carbs: 5g     Proteins: 8g     Fat: 17g

Main meals

# EASY TOFU PAD THAI

## DIRECTIONS

- Heat a small pan over medium temperature. Add tamarind, coconut aminos, coconut sugar, bean sprouts, garlic sauce, lime juice, and vegetarian fish sauce (optional).
- Cook for 30 seconds, mixing every now and then. Set aside.
- Prepare all stir fry ingredients, including cubed tofu, chopped green onions, minced garlic, bean sprouts, and chopped peanuts. Prepare also the peanut sauce in this phase (optional).
- Add Pad Thai noodles to a large bowl and bring to a boil.
- Stir and cover and cook according to package instructions (usually about 6 minutes).
- Drain noodles and toss with some sesame oil. Set aside.
- Heat a large skillet over medium heat. When hot, add oil and tofu and sauté for around 5 minutes, turning every now and then.
- Add red pepper flakes or Thai chilies, garlic, and coconut aminos.
- Mix until garlic is slightly browned.
- Add noodles, Pad Thai sauce, bean sprouts, green onions, and peanuts and cook at medium-high temperature for around 2-3 minutes.
- Plate with extra garnishes (for example: lime wedges, bean sprouts, peanut sauce, cilantro, and sriracha).
- Store the leftovers in the fridge for around 3-4 days.

## INGREDIENTS

**SAUCE**
1 ½ tsp tamarind paste/concentrate
1/3 cup (80 ml) coconut aminos
3 ½ tbsp. (42 g) coconut sugar
1 ½ tsp chili garlic sauce
1 ½ tbsp. (22 ml) lime juice
1-2 tsp Vegetarian Fish Sauce (optional)

**STIR FRY**
1 tbsp. (15 ml) sesame oil
1 cup (100 g) cubed extra firm tofu
2 Thai red chilies (fresh or dried), chopped OR 1/2 tsp chili flakes (optional)
2 cloves garlic, minced (2 cloves yield ~1 tbsp. or 6 g)
1 tbsp. (15 ml) coconut aminos (or tamari)
1 cup (104 g) bean sprouts
1 cup (100 g) chopped green onions
1/3 cup chopped roasted salted peanuts

**NOODLES**
8 oz. (227 g) Pad Thai rice noodles

**FOR SERVING (OPTIONAL)**
Lime wedges
Bean sprouts
Peanut sauce
Shredded carrot
Cilantro
Sriracha or Chili Garlic Sauce

50 mins

4

Calories per serving: 150

Carbs: 9g

Proteins: 14g

Fat: 7g

Main meals

# CRACK CHICKEN

60 mins      6

## INGREDIENTS

- 2 lb. raw (907.18 g) chicken tenders
- 8 oz. (226.8 g) cream cheese softened
- 8 oz. (226.8 g) mozzarella cheese
- 2 scallions finely sliced
- 1 cup (28g) bacon crumbles
- 1 tsp (4.93 g) garlic powder
- 1 tsp (4.93 g) onion powder
- 1 tsp (4.93 g) dill weed
- 1 tsp (4.93 g) salt

## DIRECTIONS

- Preheat oven to 400°F (200°C).
- Spray a large cooking dish with cooking spray.
- Put the chicken strips in the cooking dish.
- Mix the cream cheese, half of mozzarella, half of scallions, half of bacon, and the seasonings.
- Spread on the remaining mozzarella, scallions, and bacon.
- Bake for 30 minutes.
- Let cool for 15 minutes and serve.

Calories per serving:     437

Carbs: 4g     Proteins: 41g     Fat: 28g

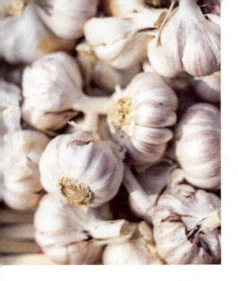
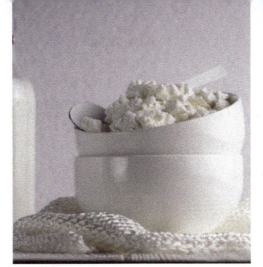
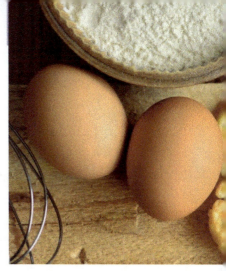

# NO NOODLE LASAGNA

 65 mins   8

## INGREDIENTS

- 1.8 cup (453.59 g) ground beef
- 2 cloves garlic minced
- 1 small onion
- 1.5 cup (369 g) ricotta cheese
- ¼ cup (50 g) Parmesan cheese
- 1 large egg use one more for a thicker lasagna
- 1 jar marinara sauce (25 oz.)
- 0.9 cup (226.8 g) mozzarella sliced

## DIRECTIONS

- Preheat the oven to 350° F (176°C). Season the ground beef with salt and pepper.
- Heat a large skillet over medium heat. Add the beef and cook until browned.
- Transfer the beef to the bottom of a 9x9 " baking pan.
- Spread the ricotta on top, then add the Parmesan.
- Pour the marinara sauce over the layers and finish off with the mozzarella.
- Cook for 30 minutes.
- Serve.

Calories per serving:     494

Carbs: 12g    Proteins: 41g    Fat: 27g

Main meals

# GINGER LIME CHICKEN

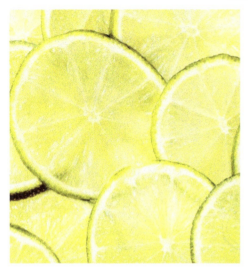

 30 mins

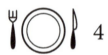 4

Calories per serving: 150

Carbs: 5g

Proteins: 20g

Fat: 6g

### INGREDIENTS

- 1½ lb. (650 g) chicken breasts, skinless
- ¼ cup (60 ml) tamari soy sauce or coconut aminos
- 2 tbsp. (30 ml) fresh lime juice
- 2 tsp (10 ml) toasted sesame oil
- 1 tsp (5 ml) lime zest
- 1 tsp (2 g) fresh ginger, grated
- 1 p" chili flakes, extra for garnish
- 1 tsp (3 g) sesame seeds, toasted, for garnish (optional)
- 1 tbsp. fresh cilantro, chopped, for garnish (optional)

### DIRECTIONS

- Place the chicken breasts in a large shallow bowl. Make holes in the chicken using a fork. This will enable the chicken to retain the marinade.
- Add soy sauce, lime juice, sesame oil, lime zest, ginger and chili flakes to a little bowl and mix. Pour the mixture over the chicken and let marinate in the fridge for at least 3 hours.
- Heat a large barbecue skillet over medium-high temperature. The, add the chicken.
- Cook for 10 to 15 minutes.
- Garnish with chili flakes, sesame seeds, and cilantro before serving.

Main meals

# BRESAOLA PLATE

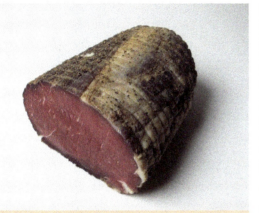

### INGREDIENTS

- 2 oz. (50 ml) bresaola, thinly sliced
- 1 oz. (30 g) (50 ml) parmesan cheese, thinly sliced
- 1 cup (225 ml) arugula lettuce
- 1 boiled large egg, cut in half
- 1 tbsp. (15 ml) fresh lemon juice
- 2 tbsp. (30 ml) olive oil
- salt and pepper to taste

### DIRECTIONS

- Layout the bresaola on the plate.
- Add arugula, parmesan cheddar, and boiled egg.
- Drizzle with olive oil, lemon juice, and add salt and pepper to taste.

 25 mins

 1

Calories per serving:    151

Carbs: 0g    Proteins: 32g    Fat: 3g

Main meals

# TURKEY WITH CREAM-CHEESE SAUCE

30 mins         4

## INGREDIENTS

- 2 tbsp. (30 ml) butter
- 1½ lb. (650 g) turkey breast
- 2 cup (475 ml) crème fraîche or heavy whipping cream
- 7 oz. (200 g) cream cheese
- 1 tbsp. (15 ml) tamari soy sauce
- salt and pepper, to taste
- 1½ oz. (40 g) small capers

Calories per serving: 815

Carbs: 7g

Proteins: 47g

Fat: 67g

## DIRECTIONS

- Preheat oven to 350°F (175°C).
- Melt ½ butter over medium temperature in a large oven proof frying pan. Season the turkey as you prefer and fry until golden brown.
- Cook turkey breasts in the oven for 15 minutes; place on a plate, and cover with foil.
- Add whipping cream and cream cheese into a small pot. Mix and bring to a boil. Lower the heat and let stew until thickened. Add soy sauce, season with salt and pepper.
- Heat remaining butter in a medium frying pan over high temperature. Sauté the capers until crispy.
- Serve turkey with sauce and fried capers.

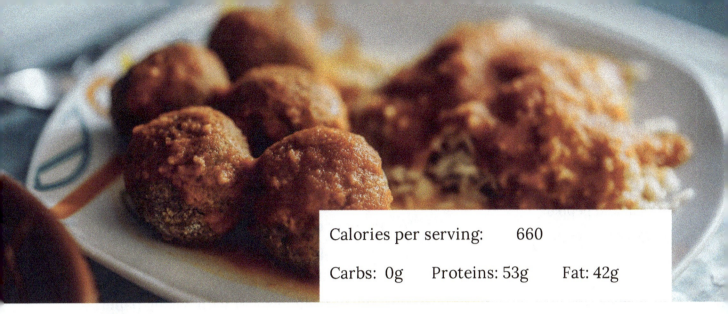

Calories per serving: 660

Carbs: 0g   Proteins: 53g   Fat: 42g

# PIMIENTO CHEESE MEATBALLS

 45 mins    4

## INGREDIENTS

- Pimiento cheese
- 1/3 cup (75 ml) mayonnaise
- ¼ cup (60 ml) pimientos or pickled jalapeños
- 1 tsp (5 ml) paprika powder or chili powder
- 1 tbsp. (15 ml) Dijon mustard
- 1 p" cayenne pepper
- 4 oz. (110 g) (225 ml) cheddar cheese, grated
- Meatballs
- 1 ½ lb. (650 g) ground beef
- 1 egg
- salt and pepper
- 2 tbsp. (30 ml) butter, for frying

## DIRECTIONS

- Start by mixing all the ingredients for the pimiento cheese in a large bowl.
- Add ground beef and the egg to the cheddar mixture. Use a wooden spoon or clean hands to combine.
- Add salt and pepper to taste.
- Make big meatballs and fry them in butter or oil in a skillet over medium temperature until they are completely cooked.
- Serve with a side dish of your choice, for example, a plate of mixed greens, and homemade mayonnaise.

Main meals

# GOAT CHEESEBURGER WITH ZUCCHINI FRIES

### SPICY TOMATO MAYONNAISE
- 1 cup (225 ml) mayonnaise
- 1 tbsp. (15 ml) tomato paste
- 1 p" cayenne pepper
- salt and pepper

### ZUCCHINI FRIES
- 1 zucchini
- 1 1/3 cup (325 ml) (150 g) almond flour
- 1 1/3 cup (325 ml) (100 g) shredded Parmesan cheese
- 1 tsp onion powder
- 1 tsp salt
- ½ tsp pepper
- 2 eggs
- 3 tbsp. (50 ml) olive oil

### BURGER
- 2 tbsp. (30 ml) butter or olive oil
- 2 red onions, thinly sliced
- 1 tbsp. (15 ml) red wine vinegar
- 1½ lb. (640 g) ground beef
- salt and pepper
- 4 oz. (100 g) goat cheese
- 3 oz. (75 g) (500 ml) lettuce

40 mins          4

### DIRECTIONS
- Preheat oven to 400°F (200°C).
- Mix all elements for the tomato mayonnaise and put them aside in the fridge.
- Cover a baking sheet with baking paper.
- Cut the zucchini lengthwise and remove the seeds.
- Break the eggs in a bowl and whisk to combine.
- Combine almond flour, parmesan cheese, onion powder, salt, and pepper in a bowl.
- Toss the zucchini in the flour, and then cover them in the eggs. Add another cover of flour.
- Place the fries on the baking sheet and shower olive oil on top. Prepare in the broiler for 20-25 minutes or until golden brown.
- Prepare the burgers. Sauté the onions in spread on medium temperature. Add the vinegar at the end; stir until creamy. Add salt and pepper to taste. Set aside.
- Shape the burger patties and fry or grill them, as you prefer.
- Season with salt and pepper.
- Place the burgers on a bed of lettuce and the onion mixture.
- Place the goat cheese on top.

*Serve with zucchini fries and tomato mayonnaise.*

Calories per serving:     87

Carbs: 4g     Proteins: 10g     Fat: 3g

Main meals

# HAMBURGER PATTIES WITH CREAMY TOMATO SAUCE AND FRIED CABBAGE

## HAMBURGER PATTIES

- 1½ lb. (650 g) ground beef
- 1 egg
- 3 oz. (75 g) crumbled feta cheese
- 1 tsp salt
- ¼ tsp ground black pepper
- 2 oz. (50 g) (200 ml) fresh parsley, finely chopped
- 1 tbsp. (15 ml) olive oil, for frying
- 2 tbsp. butter, for frying

## GRAVY

- ¾ cup (175 ml) heavy whipping cream
- 2 tbsp. (8 g) fresh parsley, coarsely chopped
- 2 tbsp. (30 ml) tomato paste or ajvar relish
- salt and pepper

## FRIED GREEN CABBAGE

- 1 ½ lb. (650 g) shredded green cabbage
- 4 ½ oz. (125 g) butter
- salt and pepper

60 mins     3

## DIRECTIONS

- Cheeseburger patties and sauce
- Add all the ingredients for the cheeseburgers to a large bowl. Mix it using a wooden spoon or your hands. Shape eight patties.
- Add butter and olive oil to a large grill.
- Fry over medium-high heat for 10 minutes, flipping them a couple of times while cooking.
- In a small bowl, mix the tomato paste and cream. Pour the mixture to the skillet when the patties are almost done.
- Mix and let stew for a couple of moments. Salt and pepper to taste.
- Sprinkle chopped parsley on top before serving.
- Margarine seared green cabbage
- Shred the cabbage finely using a food processor or a sharp blade.
- Add butter to a large skillet.
- Place the skillet over medium-high heat and sauté the cabbage for 15 minutes.
- Stir regularly and lower the heat towards the end.
- Add salt and pepper to taste.

Calories per serving: 923

Carbs: 10g

Proteins: 42g

Fat: 78g

Main meals

# OVEN-BAKED PAPRIKA CHICKEN WITH RUTABAGA

### INGREDIENTS

55 mins

4

- 2 lb. (900 g) chicken thighs (bone-in with skin) or chicken drumsticks
- 2 lb. (900 g) rutabaga or celery root, peeled and cut into 2" (5 cm) pieces
- 1 tbsp. paprika powder
- salt and pepper
- ¼ cup (60ml) olive oil
- Garlic and paprika mayo
- 1 cup (225ml) mayonnaise
- 1 tsp garlic powder
- 1 tsp paprika powder
- salt and pepper, to taste

### DIRECTIONS

- Preheat oven to 400°F (200°C).
- Place the chicken and the rutabaga in a baking dish. Season with salt, pepper, and paprika powder.
- Sprinkle with olive oil and mix well.
- Bake the chicken for 40 minutes.
- Add the mayonnaise and rutabaga to the chicken and serve.

Calories per serving: 349

Carbs: 1g   Proteins: 50g   Fat: 15g

Main meals

# CARAMELIZED ONION AND BACON PORK CHOPS

## INGREDIENTS

- 4 oz. (110 g) bacon, chopped
- 1 yellow onion, thinly sliced
- ¼ tsp salt
- ¼ tsp pepper
- 4 pork chops
- ½ cup (125 ml) beef broth
- ¼ cup (60 ml) heavy whipping cream

## DIRECTIONS

- In a large skillet, cook bacon over medium temperature.
- With a spoon, move to a bowl, and hold bacon oil.
- Add onion to bacon oil and season with salt and pepper.
- Cook, mixing regularly, for 15 to 20 minutes. Then, add onions to bacon in the bowl.
- Increase temperature to medium-high and sprinkle pork chops with salt and pepper. Add chops to skillet and cook for 3 minutes. Lower heat to medium, flip side and cook for around 7 to 10 additional minutes. Move to a dish and tent with foil.
- Add cream and stew until the mixture is thickened, for 2 or 3 minutes. Put onions and bacon to the dish and combine.
- Top pork hacks with onion and bacon and serve.

55 mins          4

Calories per serving:   130

Carbs: 1g    Proteins: 23g    Fat: 5g

Main meals

# TEX-MEX CASSEROLE

40 mins         3

### INGREDIENTS

- 1½ lb. (650 g) ground beef
- 3 oz. (75 g) butter
- 3 tbsp. Tex-Mex seasoning
- 1 cup (225 ml) (225 g) crushed tomatoes
- 2 oz. (50 g) pickled jalapeños
- 2 cup (475 ml) (225 g) shredded cheese, for example Monterey Jack
- For serving
- ¾ cup (175ml) sour cream or crème fraîche
- 1 scallion, finely chopped
- 5 oz. (150 g) (650 ml) leafy greens or iceberg lettuce
- 1 cup (225ml) guacamole (optional)

### DIRECTIONS

- Preheat oven to 400°F (200°C).
- Fry the ground beef over medium-high temperature until well cooked.
- Add Tex-Mex seasoning and crushed tomatoes.
- Mix and let rest for 5 minutes. Taste to check if it needs extra salt and pepper.
- Place the ground beef mixture in a lubed cooking dish (around 9" or 23). Pour jalapeños and cheddar.
- Bake for 15–20 minutes until golden brown on top.
- Mix the scallion with the crème fraîche or sour cream in a different bowl.
- You can serve the dish still hot with guacamole, and a portion of mixed greens.

Calories per serving:     864

Carbs: 7g     Proteins: 50g     Fat: 70g

Main meals

# CHICKEN GARAM MASALA

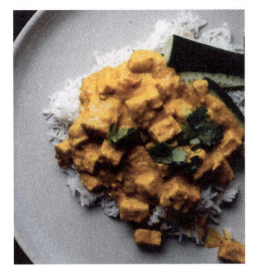

### GARAM MASALA
- 1 tsp ground cumin
- 1 tsp coriander seed, ground
- 1 tsp ground cardamom (green)
- 1 tsp turmeric, ground
- 1 tsp ground ginger
- 1 tsp paprika powder
- 1 tsp chili powder
- 1 p" ground nutmeg

### CHICKEN
- 1 lb. (450 g) chicken breasts (without skin)
- 3 tbsp. (50 ml) butter
- salt
- ½ red bell pepper, finely diced
- 1¼ cup (300 ml) unsweetened coconut cream or heavy whipping cream
- 1 tbsp. (4 g) fresh parsley, finely chopped

 50 mins

 4

## DIRECTIONS
- Preheat oven to 350°F (175°C).
- Mix the ingredients for garam masala.
- Cut the chicken breasts lengthwise. Place a large skillet over medium-high temperature and fry the chicken in butter until golden brown.
- Add the garam masala mixture to the dish and mix.
- Season with salt, and place the chicken in a baking dish.
- Add the finely diced bell pepper to a small bowl with the coconut cream and the remaining garam masala mixture.
- Pour over the chicken. Cook in the oven for around 20 minutes.
- Garnish with parsley and serve.

Calories per serving: 158

Carbs: 5g

Proteins: 21g

Fat: 5g

Main meals

## SKILLET PIZZA

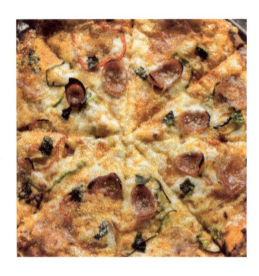

25 mins         2

### INGREDIENTS

- ½ cup (125 ml) (60 g) mozzarella cheese, shredded
- 2 oz. (50 g) fresh sausage, cooked and crumbled
- 1 oz. (30 g) pepperoni, in slices
- 1 oz. (30 g) green bell peppers, in slices
- ½ tsp Italian seasoning
- 2 tbsp. (30 ml) unsweetened tomato sauce

### DIRECTIONS

- Heat a 7" (18 cm) non-stick skillet over medium temperature.
- Sprinkle 3/4 of the cheddar on the skillet and allow melt.
- Lower the heat and cover the softened cheddar with tomatoes, sausage, green bell pepper, mozzarella, and pepperoni. Cook at low temperature for 3-4 minutes.
- Sprinkle the Italian seasoning over the pizza. The pizza is done when the cheddar on top is melted.
- Remove from heat and let cool for 5 minutes before serving.

Calories per serving:     521

Carbs: 10g    Proteins: 30g    Fat: 40g

Main meals

# CELERY & BLUE CHEESE SOUP

### INGREDIENTS

- 300 g Grated Zucchini (about 2 Zucchini)
- Heaping 1 1/2 cup (180 g) Almond Flour
- ½ cup (48 g) Coconut Flour
- 3 tbsp. (27 g) Confectioners Swerve
- 2 tsp (9 g) Baking Powder
- 1 tsp (4 g) Apple Pie Spice Mix
- 1/3 tsp Salt
- 4 Eggs, Beaten
- 3 tbsp. (42 g) Melted Butter
- 1/4 cup (59 ml) Heavy Cream
- 1 tsp (4 g) Pure Vanilla Extract
- Optional: 70 g Chopped Walnuts or Pecans for the inside and top.

75 mins    10 slices

### DIRECTIONS

- Preheat oven to 350°F (177°C). Line a 9×5″ skillet with a parchment paper.
- Grate the zucchini and wrap them in a kitchen towel, squeezing out the liquid.
- In a large bowl, mix almond flour, coconut flour, swerve, baking powder, and salt.
- Stir in beaten eggs, vanilla, heavy cream, and melted butter.
- Add zucchini and chopped pecans; blend well.
- Transfer the batter into the prepared baking sheet and sprinkle with nuts.
- Bake for 50 to 70 minutes-

NOTE: *The bread can turn brown quickly, so you should cover it with foil.*

- Once it is ready, let cool for 20 minutes, then cut..

Calories per serving:     148

Carbs: 6g     Proteins: 3g     Fat: 12g

Main meals

# THAI FISH CURRY

30 mins

4

### INGREDIENTS

- 2 oz. (50 g) coconut oil for greasing the baking dish
- 1½ lb. (650 g) salmon, boneless fillets or white fish, in pieces
- salt and pepper
- 2 oz. (50 g) butter or ghee
- 2 tbsp. red curry paste or green curry paste
- 2 cup (475 ml) canned, unsweetened coconut cream
- ½ cup (125 ml) fresh cilantro, chopped
- 1 lb. (450 g) cauliflower or broccoli

### DIRECTIONS

- Preheat oven to 400°F (200°C). Oil a medium-sized cooking dish.
- Place the fish pieces in the cooking dish. Salt and pepper to taste and put a tbsp. of butter or ghee on each fish.
- Mix coconut cream, curry paste, and chopped cilantro in a small blow and put the fish in.
- Cook in the oven for 20 minutes.
- Meanwhile, cut the cauliflower into small florets and boil in salted water for 2-3 minutes.
- Serve with the fish.

Calories per serving: 312

Carbs: 13g    Proteins: 36g    Fat: 35g

Main meals

# CHICKEN ALFREDO

25 mins    3

## INGREDIENTS

- 15.87 oz. (450 g) chicken breasts
- 3.52 oz. (100 g) mushrooms
- 0.35 oz. (10 g) garlic
- 3.38 oz. (100 ml) heavy cream
- 0.18 oz. (5 g) parsley
- Salt & Pepper to taste
- 1 tbsp. avocado oil
- 1 tbsp. butter

## DIRECTIONS

- Season the chicken with salt and pepper on both sides. Cut the mushrooms and finely chop the parsley.
- Heat the avocado oil in a skillet, then add the chicken and cook for around 3-4 minutes on each side until golden brown.
- In another skillet, add the butter and sauté the garlic.
- Add mushrooms, season with salt and pepper, and blend.
- Cook for around 3-4 min till the mushrooms release their water. Pour the heavy cream and mix well.
- Place the chicken in the skillet with the sauce and garnish with parsley.
- Serve.

Calories per serving: 720

Carbs: 28g    Proteins: 14g    Fat: 20g

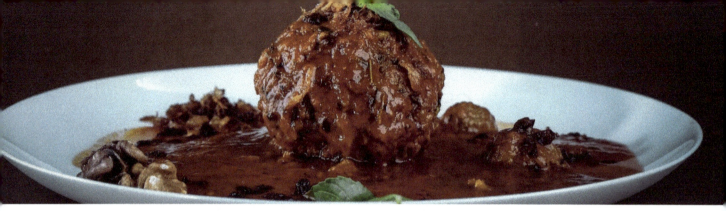

 6 servings (3 meatballs per serving)

## EASY SWEDISH MEATBALLS

Calories per 3 meatballs: 544

Carbs: 1g    Proteins: 28g    Fat: 46g

30 mins

### INGREDIENTS

- 1 lb. (453.59 g) ground pork
- 1 lb. (453.59 g) ground chuck
- 1 cup (124 g) zucchini grated (or 1 med zucchini)
- 1 egg
- 1 tsp (4.93 g) all-purpose seasoning
- 1/4 (1.23 g) tsp salt
- 2 tbsp. (29.57 g) butter
- 1 cup (235 ml) chicken broth
- 1 tbsp. (14.79 g) mustard
- 3/4 cup (178.5 ml) heavy cream

### DIRECTIONS

- Beat ground meat into a large bowl.
- With a medium grater, shred zucchini until you have around 1 stuffed cup full (don't dry or eliminate water).
- Add grated zucchini to the bowl with egg and salt.
- Mix with hands until combined.
- Melt butter in a cast iron skillet.
- Roll meat into 18 balls and place in skillet.
- Cook for around 3-5 minutes, then flip and cook another 3-5 minutes until softly seared.
- Whisk together broth, mustard, and heavy cream. Then, pour into skillet with meatballs and cook for additional 5-10 minutes.

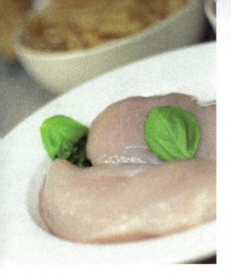
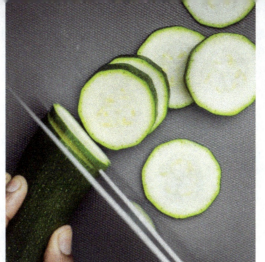
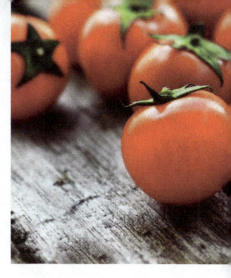

# EASY CHICKEN CHOW MEIN

 15 mins

 4

- 2 tbsp. (30 ml) peanut oil
- 160 oz. (500 g) Lilydale Free Range Chicken Thigh, thinly sliced
- 8 oz. (250 g) broccoli, cut into florets
- 4 garlic cloves, thinly sliced
- 1 long fresh red chili, deseeded, finely chopped
- extra fresh chili, finely chopped, to serve
- 1/4 small red cabbage, sliced
- 8 oz. (250 g) zucchini noodles
- 2 cup trimmed bean sprouts
- 1/2 cup roasted unsalted cashew nuts
- 2 tbsp. (30 ml) gluten-free soy sauce
- 2 tsp (10 ml) sesame oil
- Fresh coriander sprigs, to serve

## DIRECTIONS

- Heat half nut oil in a large pan at high temperature. Sauté the chicken for 2-3 minutes until golden brown.
- Move to a plate.
- Heat the remaining nut oil in the pan. Sauté broccoli, garlic, and bean sprouts for 2 minutes.
- Add the cabbage and zucchini noodles. Pan-fry for 1 minute.
- Place the chicken in the pan again together with bean sprouts, soy sauce, and sesame oil. Sauté for 1 minute.
- Serve with coriander and additional bean sprouts.

Calories per serving: 200

Carbs: 9g    Proteins: 20g    Fat: 9g

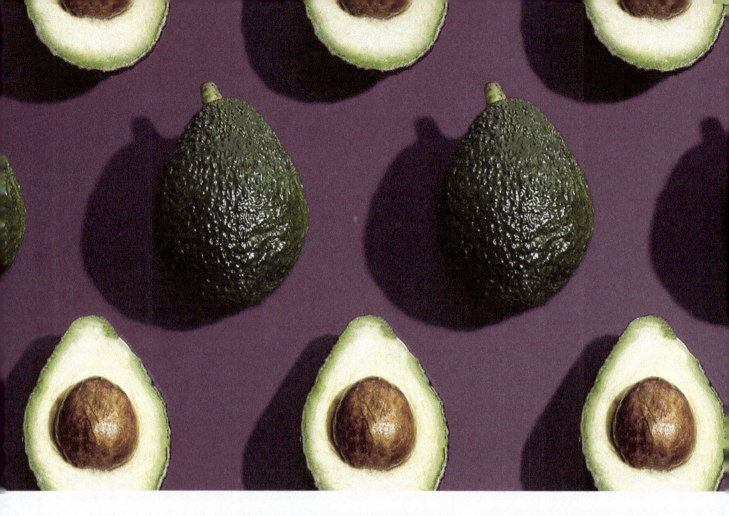

# KETO SNACKS

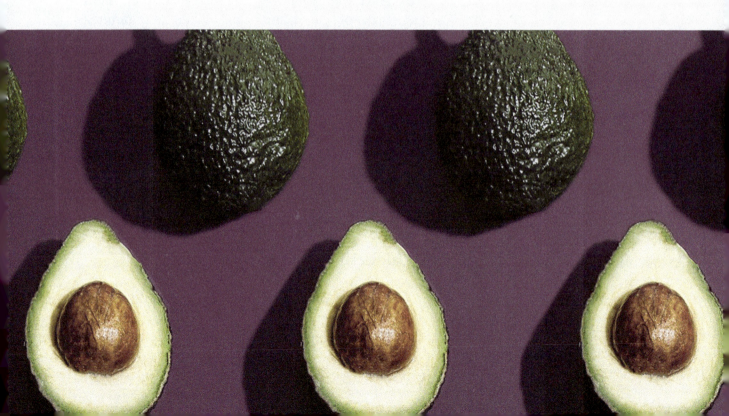

Keto Snacks

# STUFFED & GRILLED VEGETABLE BITES

45 minutes

4

## INGREDIENTS

- 1 large aubergine (about 350g/12oz)
- 1 large courgette (about 300g/11oz)
- 2 flame-roasted peppers, from a jar
- 1 garlic clove, crushed
- 3 tbsp. (50 ml) olive oil
- 250 g (1 cup) tub ricotta
- 25 g (1 oz.) finely grated parmesan (or vegetarian alternative)
- 3 sundried or semi-dried tomatoes in oil (from a jar), drained and finely chopped
- finely grated zest 0.5 lemon
- 8 basil leaves
- small handful parsley, leaves picked and roughly chopped
- ½ tsp (2.5 ml) paprika

## DIRECTIONS

- Cut the aubergine and courgette into slim pieces around 2-3mm thick – you ought to have 8 cuts of each. Wash the peppers, remove any seeds and cut into quarters. Mix the garlic with the olive oil and flavorings.
- Heat a frying pan over medium temperature. Brush the vegetable cuts with the garlic oil and cook for 2-3 min each side. You could also use a grill.
- Set aside on a plate and let cool.
- Mix the cheese, tomatoes, and lemon zest. Spread out the cuts of aubergine on a plate. Top each with a cut of courgette, pepper, and a basil leaf. Pour 1 tbsp. of the cheddar mixture on top and roll the vegetables up.
- Assemble the skewers.
- For the final touch, top with parsley leaves and paprika.

Calories per serving: 110

Carbs: 8g     Proteins: 6g     Fat: 8g

Keto Snacks

# ULTIMATE GUACAMOLE

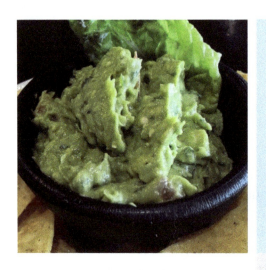

### INGREDIENTS
- 1 small (125 g) (4 ½ oz.) red onion
- 1 medium (100 g) overripe tomato
- 1 red chili, deseeded
- 1 large handful fresh coriander
- 1 lime
- 3 large or 4 medium (150 g) ripe avocados
- olive oil

 25 mins

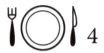 4

### DIRECTIONS
- In a food processor, beat the onion, tomato, and the coriander until finely chopped (you can also do this by hand); then, move to a bowl.
- Squeeze the lime into the mixture.
- Cut your avocados in half, remove the pit and scoop out the smooth part with a spoon.
- With clean hands, squash the avocado to a puree to make it creamy. Save a couple of pieces for a touch on the surface.
- Serve right away with olive oil on top and some more coriander.

Calories per serving: 51

Carbs: 3g

Proteins: 1g

Fat: 4g

## AVOCADO WITH TAMARI & GINGER DRESSING

5 mins      2

### INGREDIENTS

- 1 small garlic clove, shredded
- ½ tsp (2.5 ml) shredded ginger
- 1 tsp (5 ml) tamari
- 2 tsp (10 ml) lemon juice
- 1 avocado

### DIRECTIONS

- Blend the garlic, ginger, tamari, and lemon juice in a small bowl.
- Dilute with 1-2 tsp water.
- Cut the avocado in half and add the mixture.
- Eat with a spoon!

Calories per serving: 131

Carbs: 10g    Proteins: 2g    Fat: 10g

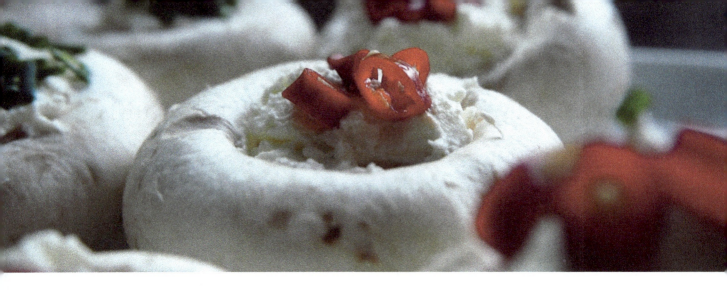

# CHEESY AUTUMN MUSHROOMS

 15 mins  4

## INGREDIENTS

- 4 large field mushrooms
- 100 g (1/2 cup) gorgonzola or other blue cheese, crumbled
- 25 g (1/8 cup) walnuts, toasted and roughly chopped
- 4 thyme sprigs
- knob butter, cut into small pieces
- rocket leaves, to serve

## DIRECTIONS

- Preheat oven to 200°F/180°C. Arrange the mushrooms on a cooking dish. Spread over the cheddar, pecans, and thyme sprigs.
- Put in the oven and cook for 10 min until the cheddar is melted. Set some rocket leaves on a dish and put the mushrooms on top.

Calories per serving: 181

Carbs: 1g   Proteins: 9g   Fat: 16g

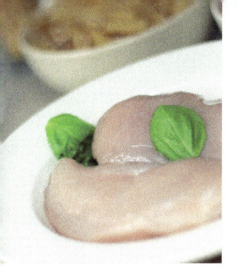
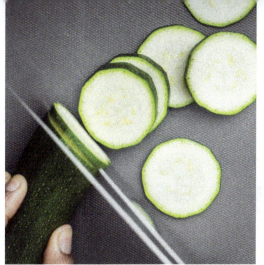
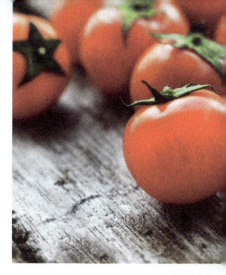

## KETO SNACK BOX

 5 mins      2 containers

### INGREDIENTS

- 6 pieces of sliced turkey breast (3 pieces per container)
- 2 hard-boiled egg, cut in half
- 1 cup (250 g) cherry tomato, cut in half
- 1 cup (250 g) diced cucumber
- 1 cup (250 g) cubed mild cheddar cheese

### DIRECTIONS

- Add turkey, egg, tomatoes, cucumber, and 1/2 cup cheddar in a food container.
- Store in the fridge until ready to eat.

Calories per serving:     230

Carbs: 5g     Proteins: 13g     Fat: 17g

Keto Snacks

# MEXICAN EGG ROLL

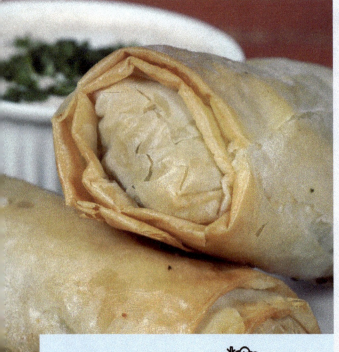

### DIRECTIONS

- Beat the egg.
- Heat some oil in a medium non-stick skillet.
- Add the egg and whirl around the skillet, like you were making a pancake, and cook until set. It is not necessary to flip it.
- Move the batter to a plate, spread with tomato salsa, sprinkle with coriander.
- Serve it right away – you can save it for 2 days in the fridge.

### INGREDIENTS

- 1 large egg
- a little rapeseed oil for frying
- 2 tbsp. (30 ml) tomato salsa
- 1 tbsp. (15 ml) fresh coriander

2

15 minutes

Calories per serving: 180

Carbs: 6g  Proteins: 20g  Fat: 8g

Keto Snacks

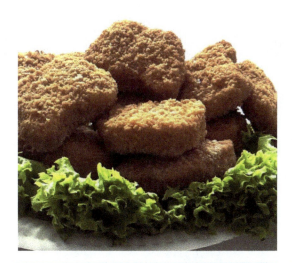

## CAULIFLOWER TOTS

30 mins          10-15

### INGREDIENTS

- 1 large head of cauliflower cut into florets
- 1 cup (250 g) of shredded cheese like cheddar or mozzarella
- 2 eggs
- 2 tbsp. (30 ml) freshly chopped Italian flat-leaf parsley
- ½ tsp (2 ml) smoked paprika
- ¼ (1 ml) tsp cayenne pepper
- 1 (5ml) tsp olive oil
- Kosher salt & pepper
- Non-stick spray

### DIRECTIONS

- Preheat oven to 400°F (200°C)
- In a food processor, rice the cauliflower florets.
- Place the cauliflower in a microwave container, add some water and microwave for 5 minutes.
- When the cauliflower is cool enough, place in a kitchen towel and squeeze to remove half of the water.
- Place in a large bowl, stir in the remaining ingredients (except the non-stick spray), and mix well.
- Using a cookie scoop, measure out the mixture. Then, shape in your hands.
- Spray the tots with non-stick spray.
- Cook for 20 minutes, flipping the tots over at half time.
- Serve straight away.

Calories per serving:     29

Carbs: 1g     Proteins: 2g     Fat: 2g

Keto Snacks

# SALAMI CHIPS

8 hrs 10 mins

4

## INGREDIENTS

- 2 wooden skewers
- 10 oz. (100 g) Salami sliced thin
- 1/3 cup (80 g) Franks Hot Sauce

## DIRECTIONS

- Pour the Franks Hot Sauce into a bowl.
- Take each cut of Salami and scoop it in the hot sauce until completely covered.
- Place uniformly in a food dehydrator and set to high.
- Let dehydrate for 8-10 hrs.
- Note: Time may vary depending on type of salami, room temperature, and quantity of sauce, so check regularly.
- Once completely dry, place in a bowl and serve.

Calories per serving: 507

Carbs: 3g   Proteins: 25g   Fat: 44g

Keto Snacks

# PROTEIN BALLS

## INGREDIENTS

- 1 cup (250 g) Hemp Hearts
- 1/2 (120 g) cup shredded unsweetened coconut
- 1/2 cup (120 g) almond slices
- 1/4 cup (38 g) chia seeds
- 1/4 cup (38 g) flaxseed
- 1/2 cup (120 g) peanut butter
- 2 tbsp. (1 oz. or 30 ml) ChocZero syrup
- 2 tbsp. (1 oz. or 30 ml) vanilla extract
- 1/4 cup (38g) ChocZero milk chocolate chips

## DIRECTIONS

- In a large bowl, combine all the ingredients.
- Scoop out a tbsp. size portion of the mixture and put on a baking sheet.
- Let cool in the fridge for about an hour to solidify; then serve.

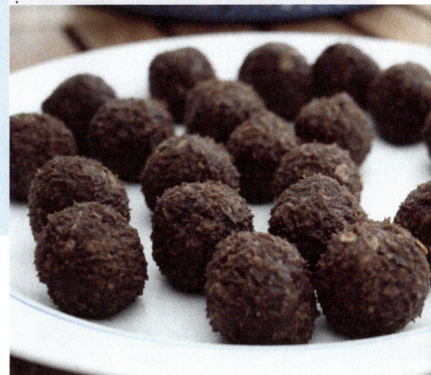

5 mins        24

Calories per serving:      252

Carbs: 4g      Proteins: 12g      Fat: 19g

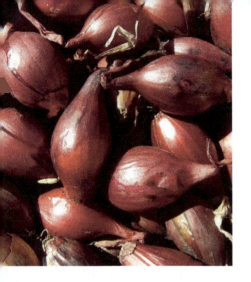 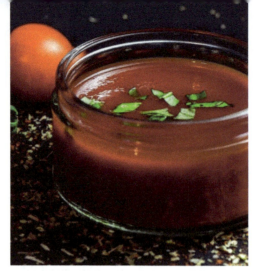 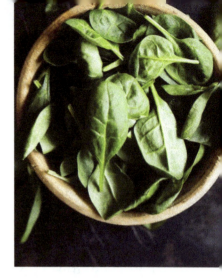

## BACON BUTTER

 15 mins   4

### INGREDIENTS

- 4½ oz. (125 g) butter, at room temperature
- 2 shallots, finely chopped
- 2 oz. (50 g) bacon, finely chopped
- 1 tbsp. fresh basil, finely chopped
- 1 tsp tomato paste

### DIRECTIONS

- Fry shallots and bacon in 1 tbsp. of butter for around 5 minutes.
- Let cool and combine with the remaining butter, tomato paste, and basil.
- Add salt and pepper to taste.
- Store in a small bowl and put in the fridge for about 30 minutes, so it solidifies.

Calories per serving:    35

Carbs: 0g    Proteins: 3g    Fat: 3g

Keto Snacks

# GARLIC BREAD

1 hr 35 mins

8

### INGREDIENTS

- 1 ½ (7 g) sachet instant dried yeast
- 1 tbsp. (15 ml) pouring cream
- 80ml (1/3 cup) warm water
- 155 g (1 1/2 cup) almond meal
- 2 tbsp. (30 ml) psyllium husk
- 1 tbsp. (15 ml) ground flaxseed
- 1 tsp (5 ml) baking powder
- 1/2 tsp (2 ml) table salt
- 3 eggs, lightly whisked
- 2 tbsp. (30 ml) olive oil
- 2 tsp (30 ml) apple cider vinegar
- 3 garlic cloves, finely chopped
- 2 tbsp. (15 ml) olive oil
- 100 g (1 cup) grated Devondale Mozzarella Cheese Block (500g)
- Chopped continental parsley to serve

### DIRECTIONS

- Line a 20 cm cooking dish with baking paper. Place yeast, cream, and water in a small bowl. Whisk to combine. Set aside for 10 minutes.
- In a large bowl, whisk together almond meal, psyllium husk, flaxseed, heating powder, and salt.
- Add the yeast blend, egg, olive oil, and vinegar. Whisk well. Move to the cooking dish. Cover with plastic wrap and Set aside for 1 hour.
- Preheat oven to 400°F (200°C).
- Cook the bread for 15 minutes.
- Sprinkle with olive oil, garlic, and grated cheese.
- Cook for additional 10 minutes until cheese is melted.
- Sprinkle with parsley and serve.

Calories per serving: 122

Carbs: 4g   Proteins: 6g   Fat: 10g

Keto Snacks

# KETO SALAD

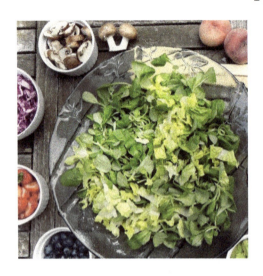

15 mins      1

### DIRECTIONS

- Dice the tomatoes and avocado. Cut the hardboiled egg.
- Place the mixed greens into a bowl or plate.
- Place tomatoes, avocado, egg, chicken, feta, and bacon on top of the greens, divided into levels.
- Serve.

### INGREDIENTS

- 4 cherry tomatoes
- ½ avocado
- 1 hardboiled egg
- 2 cup (75 g) mixed green salad
- 2 oz. (55 g) chicken breast, shredded
- 1 oz. (28 g) feta cheese, crumbled
- ¼ cup (50 g) cooked bacon, crumbled

Calories per serving:     670

Carbs: 7g     Proteins: 50g     Fat: 48g

# DESSERTS

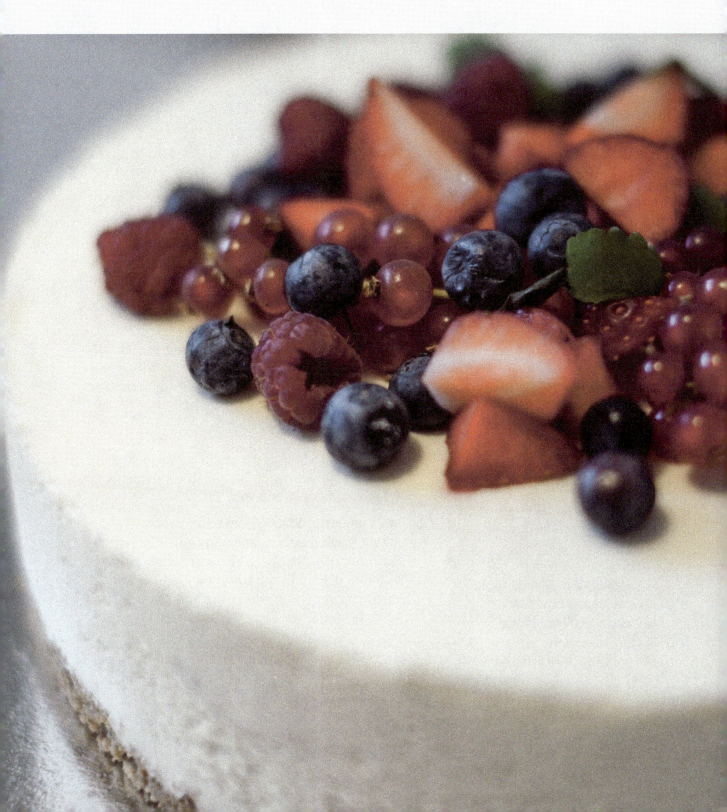

Desserts

## FRAPPUCCINO SLICE

 4 hr 10 mins  16

Calories per serving: 211

Carbs: 211g   Proteins: 0g   Fat: 22g

### INGREDIENTS

- 2 tbsp. (15 ml) boiling water
- 2 1/2 tsp (30 ml) gelatin powder
- 8oz (1 cup) (250 g) cream cheese, at room temperature, chopped
- 2 tbsp. powdered stevia
- 1/3 cup (80 ml) strong espresso coffee, cooled
- 1 tsp (5 ml) vanilla extract
- 1/2 cup (120 ml) thickened cream, whipped, plus extra, whipped, to serve
- Coffee beans, to serve (optional)
- Cacao powder, to dust
- Base
- 1 cup (100 g) pecans
- 1 1/4 cup (130 g) almond meal
- 1 tbsp. cacao powder
- 1 tbsp. powdered stevia
- 1 egg
- 2 tbsp. (30 ml unsalted butter, melted)

### DIRECTIONS

- Preheat oven to 360°F (180°C).
- Line a 16 x 26cm slice pan with baking paper. Allow the paper to overhang the two long sides.
- For the base, place the pecans in a food processor and process until finely ground.
- Add the almond meal, cacao, and stevia. Mix well, then add the egg and butter. Mix again, then move to prepared pan. Press mixture into the base.
- Bake for 10 minutes. Set aside to cool.
- Place the boiling water in a small heatproof bowl. Sprinkle over the gelatin powder and whisk until gelatin dissolves.
- With electric beaters, beat the cream cheese, stevia, cooled coffee, and vanilla in a large bowl until smooth. Beat in the gelatin blend until well combined. Fold in the whipped cream. Pour the mixture over the cooled base and use a spatula to smooth the surface.
- Cover and place in the refrigerator for 4 hours.
- With a sharp knife, cut the slice into 16 squares. Top with extra whipped cream and espresso beans (optional).
- Serve with cacao powder.

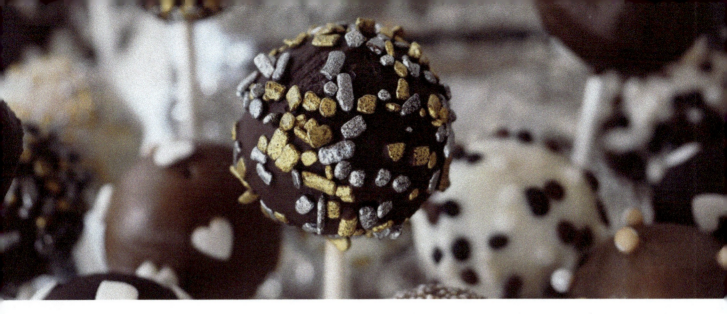

# CHOC-ORANGE BLISS BALLS

 20 mins  20

## INGREDIENTS

- 1 tbsp. chia seeds
- 300g (2 cup) macadamia nuts
- 120g (1 1/3 cup) desiccated coconut
- 2 tbsp. (30 ml) xylitol
  2 tbsp. cacao powder
- 1 tbsp. (15 ml) orange zest
- 1oz (30 g) butter, melted, cooled
- P" of sea salt

Calories per serving: 118

Carbs: 16g

Proteins: 3g

Fat: 4g

## DIRECTIONS

- Place the chia seeds and 2 tbsp. water in a bowl. Set aside for 10 minutes, blending occasionally, until water has dried up and the mixture is gel-like.
- Place the macadamias, 1 cup of the coconut, xylitol, cacao powder, orange zest, butter, chia seeds, and salt in a food processor. Process until finely chopped.
- Move the nut mixture to a bowl. Make small balls.
- Put the remaining coconut on a plate, then move balls in coconut to delicately cover.
- Serve.
- Store in in the fridge for as long as two weeks.

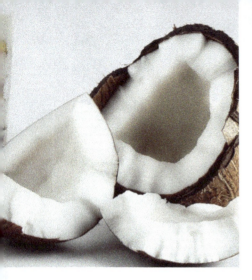 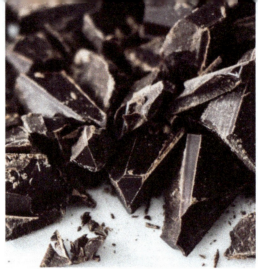 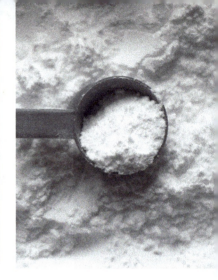

# KETO BOUNTY BARS

 15 mins    20

## INGREDIENTS

- 1 cup (200 g) of coconut flakes
- ¼ cup (50 g) of coconut oil
- 2/3 cup (100 g) of Philadelphia cream cheese full fat
- 1/3 cup (50 g) of whey or vegan protein
- 5-8 drops of vanilla

### TOPPING
- ½ (70g) dark chocolate 90%
- 1 tbsp. coconut oil
- Coconut flakes

## DIRECTIONS

- Put the coconut flakes into the oven at 360°F (180°C) for around 7 minutes until they turn bright.
- Put them into a bowl and mix with coconut oil, Philadelphia cream cheddar, whey or vegan protein, and drops of vanilla.
- Form small bars and put them on a baking sheet.
- Put them into the fridge for 30 minutes.
- As for the topping, mix the melted dark chocolate with coconut oil. Pour chocolate over the bars and sprinkle with more coconut flakes.
- Now cool them again in the refrigerator for two hours.
- Serve.
- Store in the fridge for as long as 5 days.

Calories per serving:    102

Carbs: 2g    Proteins: 1g    Fat: 10g

Desserts

# CHOCOLATE CHIP COOKIE FAT BOMBS

45 mins      30

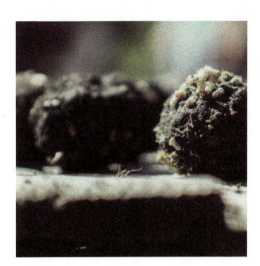

## INGREDIENTS

- 1/2 cup (120 ml) butter softened
- 1/3 cup (80 ml) Swerve confectioners' sugar (Erythritol sweetener)
- 1 tsp (5 ml) pure vanilla extract
- 1/2 tsp (2 ml) kosher salt
- 2 cup (480 ml) almond flour
- 9 oz. (240 ml) dark chocolate chips
- 8 oz. (240 g) sugar-free chocolate chips

## DIRECTIONS

- In a large bowl beat butter with a hand mixer.
- Mix in sugar, salt, and vanilla.
- Add in almond flour and mix until dough consistency forms.
- Pour in dark chocolate chips and mix. Cover with plastic wrap and place in the refrigerator for 10-15 minutes.
- Remove dough from fridge and use a cookie scoop to form 1-" balls.
- Place on a rimmed baking sheet lined with parchment paper.
- In a microwave-safe dish melt sugar-free chocolate chips for 2 minutes.
- Dip each fat bomb in melted chocolate and then put back onto the lined baking sheet.
- Place in freezer for 5 minutes.
- Serve.

Calories per serving:     137

Carbs: 12g    Proteins: 2g    Fat: 11g

Desserts

# CHOCOLATE PEANUT BUTTER PROTEIN BARS

20 mins     24

## INGREDIENTS

- 1/2 cup (60 g) coconut flour
- 3/4 cup (2 scoops) protein powder
- 2 cup (500 g) peanut butter can sub for any nut or seed butter
- 1/2 cup (112 g) maple syrup
- 2 cup (360 g) chocolate chips of choice (optional)

## DIRECTIONS

- Line a baking dish with parchment paper and put it in a safe spot.
- For thicker bars, use an 8 x 8-" dish. For thinner bars, use any size greater.
- In a large blending bowl, add your dry fixings and mix well.
- In a small blending bowl, melt your nut butter with maple syrup until combined. Add to dry fixings and blend until completely combined.
- Transfer nut butter protein bar batter into the lined baking dish and press firmly.
- Cool or freeze until solid.
- Once solid, cut into bars and cover in chocolate!

Calories per serving:     230

Carbs: 20g    Proteins: 22g    Fat: 8g

Desserts

# VANILLA MUG CAKE

2 mins

## INGREDIENTS

- 1 tbsp. (14.79 g) refined coconut oil melted
- ¼ tsp (1.23 g) vanilla
- 1 tbsp. (14.79 g) sour cream
- 1 egg
- 1.5 tbsp. (22.18 g) erythritol
- 3 tbsp. (44.36 g) almond flour
- 1 tbsp. (14.79 g) coconut flour
- ¼ tsp (1.23 g) baking powder
- tiny p" salt
- thickened cream, whipped, plus extra, whipped, to serve
- Coffee beans, to serve (optional)
- Cacao powder, to dust
- Base
- 1 cup (100 g) pecans
- 1 1/4 cup (130 g) almond meal
- 1 tbsp. cacao powder
- 1 tbsp. powdered stevia
- 1 egg
- 2 tbsp. (30 ml unsalted butter, melted)

## DIRECTIONS

- In a microwave-safe cup, mix all the ingredients well.
- Microwave it for 1 to 5 minutes.
- Serve.

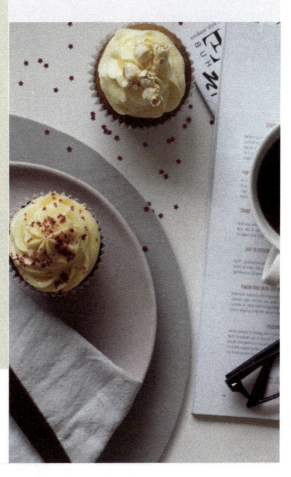

Calories per serving: 216

Carbs: 8g    Proteins: 9g    Fat: 18g

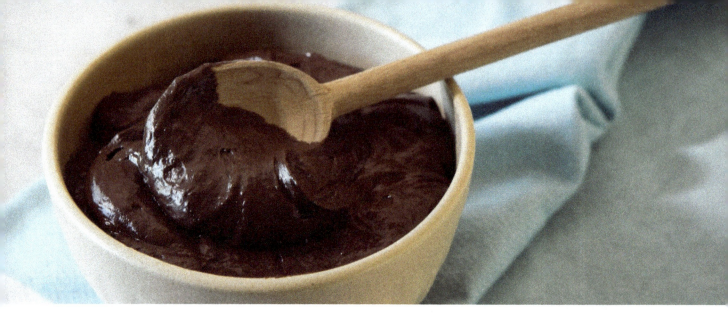

10 mins

5

# CHOCOLATE MOUSSE

## INGREDIENTS

- 1 cup (238 g) heavy whipping cream
- 1 cup (227 g) cream cheese
- ¼ cup (21.5 g) cocoa powder
- ¼ cup (45.5 g) powdered erythritol or two tbsp. of my sweetener, finely ground
- P" of sea salt

## DIRECTIONS

- Add all fixings to a large bowl. With a hand blender, beat fixings together for 2 minutes, scratch down the sides of the bowl, and keep blending for an additional 3 minutes, or until the mixture forms pinnacles and is thick and velvety.
- Taste and add extra sweetener, if desired.
- Store in lunch box in the fridge for as long as 3 days.

Calories per serving:     335

Carbs:  2g

Proteins:  2g

Fat: 37g

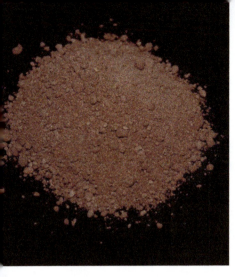
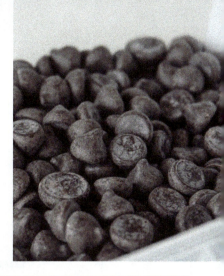

Desserts

8 mins      10

# CHOCOLATE CHAFFLE RECIPE

Calories per serving: 202

Carbs: 3g

Proteins: 16g

Fat: 13g

## INGREDIENTS

- 8 oz. (226.8 g) cream cheese
- 8 oz. (226.8 g) heavy cream
- ½ cup (100 g) powdered erythritol
- ⅓ cup (37.33 g) almond flour
- ⅓ cup (84 g) erythritol
- ¼ cup (21.5 g) cocoa powder
- 2 oz. (56.7 g) cream cheese softened
- ½ tsp baking powder
- ½ tsp vanilla
- 3 tbsp. sugar-free chocolate chips
- ½ (70g) dark chocolate 90%
- 1 tbsp. coconut oil
- Coconut flakes

## DIRECTIONS

- Grease and preheat waffle iron at medium temperature.
- Add all the wet ingredients to a blender.
- Top with the dry ingredients (except the chocolate chips).
- Mix until smooth, scratching down the sides, if needed. Mix in the chocolate chips.
- Pour around 3 tbsp. of batter onto the heated waffle iron.
- Cook until golden brown, checking regularly and paying attention not overcooking it.
- Delicately remove the waffle.
- Repeat with the remaining batter.
- Let cool for a moment and serve with your desired toppings.
- 
- Put them into the fridge for 30 minutes.
- As for the topping, mix the melted dark chocolate with coconut oil. Pour chocolate over the bars and sprinkle with more coconut flakes.
- Now cool them again in the refrigerator for two hours.
- Serve.
- Store in the fridge for as long as 5 days.

Desserts

# CHEESECAKE FLUFF

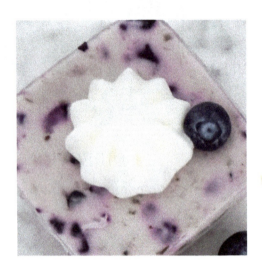

45 mins                                    4

### DIRECTIONS

- Whip the heavy cream until hardened pinnacles form. Move to a different bowl.
- Whip the cream cheese and erythritol until bright and velvety.
- Add ⅓ of the whipped cream and blend well.
- Gradually add the remaining whipped cream.
- Spoon or line into small serving bowls.

### INGREDIENTS

- 8 oz. (226.8 g) cream cheese
- 8 oz. (226.8 g) heavy cream
- ½ cup (100 g) powdered erythritol
- 
- 2 cup (480 ml) almond flour
- 9 oz. (240 ml) dark chocolate chips
- 8 oz. (240 g) sugar-free chocolate chips

Calories per serving:       330

Carbs: 3g    Proteins: 4.5g    Fat: 30.5g

Desserts

# PUMPKIN PANCAKES

30 mins

8

### BATTER
- 4 eggs
- 1 cup (210 g) cottage cheese
- 1 cup (245 g) pumpkin puree
- ¼ cup (62.5 g) almond milk
- ⅔ cup (74.67 g) almond flour
- ⅓ cup (40 g) coconut flour
- 1 tsp vanilla
- 1 tsp baking powder
- ⅓ cup (84 g) erythritol
- 1.5 tsp pumpkin pie spice

### CREAM CHEESE ICING
- 8 oz. (226.8 g) cream cheese softened
- ⅓ cup (84 g) erythritol or stevia
- Cottage Cheese Icing (optional)
- 1 cup (210 g) cottage cheese
- 2 tbsp. butter
- ¼ cup (63 g) erythritol or monk fruit extract
- ½ tsp vanilla

### DIRECTIONS
- Mix all the ingredients in the blender, placing the wet ones in first. Blend until smooth.
- Preheat a large frying pan over medium temperature.
- Spray generously with cooking spray.
- Drop tbsp. of batter onto the frying pan.
- Cook well before flipping.
- For the cream cheddar icing:
- Join the cream cheese and sweetener and blend well.

*For the cream cheese icing:*

- Mix cottage cheese until smooth in a food processor.
- Add the remaining ingredients and blend well.

Calories per serving: 110

Carbs: 2g   Proteins: 4g   Fat: 10g

## Desserts

# FRENCH TOAST CASSEROLE

### BREAD

- 3 tbsp. butter
- 3 tbsp. almond flour
- 3 tbsp. coconut flour
- 3 eggs
- ¼ cup (56.5 g) coconut milk
- 2 tsp baking powder

### CREAM CHEESE FILLING

- 8 oz. (226.8 g) cream cheese
- 2 tbsp. powdered erythritol
- 1 tsp vanilla

### CUSTARD

- 3 eggs
- 1 cup (226 g) coconut milk
- ½ cup (110 g) brown sugar sweetener
- ¼ cup (59.5 g) heavy cream
- ½ tsp cinnamon

*Topping*

- 1 cup (112 g) almond flour
- 5 tbsp. butter
- ⅓ cup (73.33 g) brown sugar sweetener
- ½ tsp cinnamon
- Sugar-free syrup optional

1 hr 15 mins     5

### DIRECTIONS

- Preheat oven to 350°F (180°C).
- Stir together ingredients for the bread. Spread in an 8x8 baking dish.
- Bake for 20-25 minutes until golden.
- Cool for 10 minutes and cut into cubes.
- Mix together the cream cheese filling.
- Mix the custard ingredients until smooth.
- Cut the butter into the flour, sweetener, and cinnamon to make crumbs for the topping.
- To assemble, place cubes of bread in the baking dish.
- Drop the cream cheese filling on top of the bread.
- Pour the custard over the top. Sprinkle on the topping.
- Bake for 40-45 minutes until golden brown and set in the middle.
- Serve with sugar-free maple syrup.

Calories per serving:    388

Carbs: 6g    Proteins: 7g    Fat: 36g

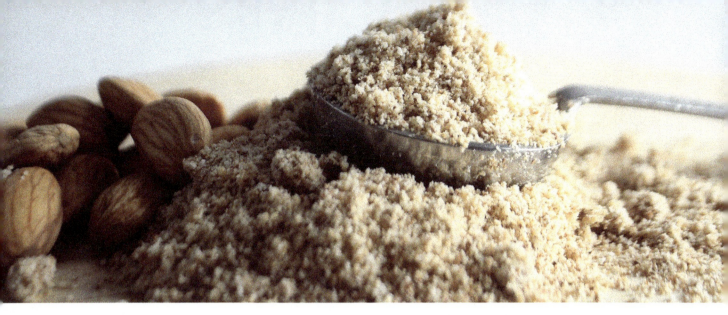

20 mins    8

# FUNFETTI COOKIE BITES

## INGREDIENTS

- 1.5 cup (168 g) almond flour
- 4 oz. (113.4 g) butter
- ¼ cup (63 g) erythritol
- 2 tsp gelatin
- ½ tsp vanilla
- ½ tsp almond extract
- ½ tsp butter extract
- 3 tbsp. sugar-free sprinkles

Calories per serving:   229
Carbs: 6g
Proteins: 3g
Fat: 14g

## DIRECTIONS

- Preheat oven to 350°F (180°C).
- Mix the dough ingredients, except the sprinkles, in the food processor.
- Process until a ball of dough forms. This should take 2-3 minutes at high speed.
- Add the sprinkles and pulse just until they are evenly distributed.
- Press into an 8x10" rectangle, ½ thick, on a material lined preparing sheet. Cut into ½" squares.
- Separate the cookies.
- Bake for 8-10 minutes or until lightly browned around the edges.
- Let cool and serve.

Desserts

# BLACKBERRY CHEESECAKE

20 mins

**Calories per serving:** 336

**Carbs:** 5g  **Proteins:** 8g  **Fat:** 32g

12

## CRUST

- 1 ½ cup (168 g) almond flour
- ⅓ cup (75.67 g) salted butter melted
- ¼ cup (63 g) erythritol
- 3 tbsp. almond butter

## FILLING

- 2 tbsp. gelatin
- 8 oz. (226.8 g) cream cheese softened
- 1 cup (210 g) cottage cheese
- ½ cup (126 g) erythritol
- ¼ cup (57.5 g) sour cream
- ½ tsp vanilla
- 2 cup (288 g) blackberries pureed and strained
- fresh blackberries to garnish (optional)
- ⅓ cup (84 g) erythritol
- ¼ cup (21.5 g) cocoa powder
- 2 oz. (56.7 g) cream cheese softened
- ½ tsp baking powder
- ½ tsp vanilla
- 3 tbsp. sugar-free chocolate chips
- ½ (70g) dark chocolate 90%
- 1 tbsp. coconut oil
- Coconut flakes

## DIRECTIONS

- To prepare the no-bake crust, blend in a food processor the crust ingredients until well combined.
- Bloom the gelatin by sprinkling it over ¼ cup of cold water.
- Let sit for 5 minutes. Mix in ¼ cup very hot water. Stir until dissolved.
- In a food processor, process the cream cheese and cottage cheese until smooth.
- Add the sour cream and vanilla. Pulse until well combined. Scrape down the sides, if needed.
- Add in half of the gelatin mixture and mix well.
- Pour ½ of the filling into the prepared crust.
- Add the blackberry puree and the remaining gelatin to the rest of the cheesecake filling. Mix well. Pour on top of the plain cheesecake and spread evenly.
- Refrigerate at least 2-3 hours.
- Serve with additional berries (optional).
- the heated waffle iron.
- Cook until golden brown, checking regularly and paying attention not overcooking it.
- Delicately remove the waffle.
- Repeat with the remaining batter.
- Let cool for a moment and serve with your desired toppings.
- Put them into the fridge for 30 minutes.
- As for the topping, mix the melted dark chocolate with coconut oil. Pour chocolate over the bars and sprinkle with more coconut flakes.
- Now cool them again in the refrigerator for two hours.
- Serve.

*Store in the fridge for as long as 5 days.*

## Desserts

# STRAWBERRY CHEESECAKE

1 hr 35 mins        12

## INGREDIENTS

- Crust
- 1.5 cup (168 g) almond flour or almond meal
- 4 tbsp. (59.15 g) salted butter melted
- 2 tbsp. (29.57 g) Trim Healthy Mama Gentle Sweet or my sweetener
- Filling
- 16 oz. (453.59 g) cream cheese
- ½ cup (115g) sour cream
- 4 eggs
- 2 tsp (9.86) vanilla
- ¾ cup (189 g) Trim Healthy Mama Gentle Sweet or my sweetener
- 1 cup (144 g) strawberries hulled
- Garnish
- 1 cup (144 g) strawberries sliced
- 2 cup (480 ml) almond flour
- 9 oz. (240 ml) dark chocolate chips
- 8 oz. (240 g) sugar-free chocolate chips

## DIRECTIONS

- Preheat oven to 350°F (180°C).
- In a food processor, combine the crust ingredients and process until well combined.
- Press into the bottom and up the sides of an 8-inch springform pan.
- Bake the crust for 10 minutes.
- Meanwhile, process the cream cheese in the food processor until smooth.
- Add the sour cream, eggs, vanilla, and sweetener. Process until well combined.
- Once the crust has partially baked, add half the filling to the crust, then put the strawberries into the food processor and blend into the rest of the filling. Drizzle over the plain cheesecake filling.
- Bake for 1 hour 20 minutes.
- Let cool for 3-4 hours before serving.

Calories per serving: 348

Carbs: 4g     Proteins: 8g     Fat: 33g

# PART 3

## 30-Day Keto Diet Meal Plan

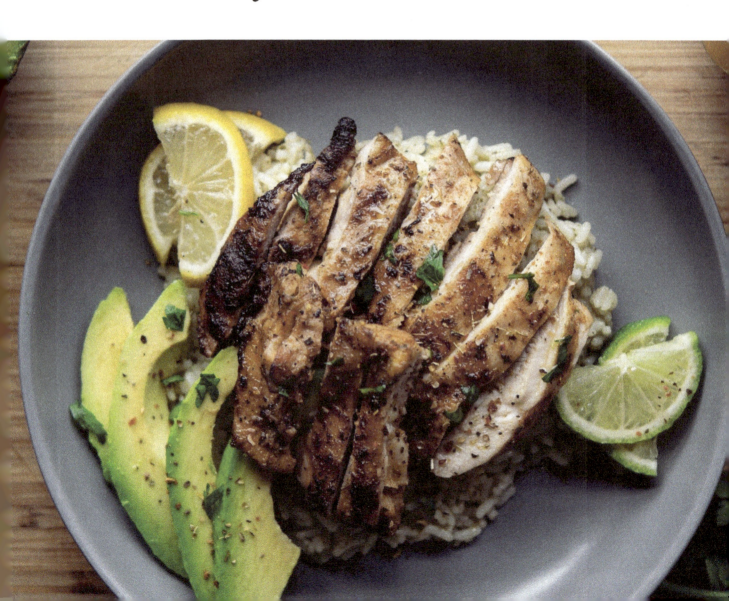

|  | Breakfast | Lunch | Dinner | Snack |
|---|---|---|---|---|
| DAY 1 | Pancakes with Berries and Whipped Cream | Thai Fish Curry | Keto Salad | Easy Banana Muffins |
| DAY 2 | Jill's Cheese-Crusted Omelette | Mexican Cauliflower Rice | Stuffed Chicken Breast with Zoodles and Tomato Sauce | Zucchini Bread |
| DAY 3 | Chocolate Pancake Cereal | Pesto Chicken Casserole with Feta Cheese and Olives | Goat Cheeseburger with Zucchini Fries | Vanilla Mug Cake |
| DAY 4 | Scrambled Eggs | Spaghetti Squash Casserole | Hamburger Patties with Creamy Tomato Sauce and Fried Cabbage | Chocolate Peanut Butter Protein Bars |
| DAY 5 | Keto Cornbread | Mexican Cauliflower Rice | Ginger Lime Chicken | Pumpkin Pancakes |
| DAY 6 | Egg Butter with Smoked Salmon and Avocado | No Noodle Lasagna | Oven-Baked Paprika Chicken with Rutabaga | Chocolate Mousse |
| DAY 7 | Keto Cornbread | Keto Salad | Caramelized Onion and Bacon Pork Chops | Funfetti Cookie Bites |
| DAY 8 | Chocolate Pancake Cereal | Easy Tofu Pad Thai | Hamburger Patties with Creamy Tomato Sauce and Fried Cabbage | Vanilla Mug Cake |
| DAY 9 | Omelet Wrap with Salmon & Avocado | Skillet Pizza | Chicken Curry Pie | Cheesecake Fluff |
| DAY 10 | Keto Cornbread | Taco Pie | Pot Barbecue Chicken | Chocolate Mousse |
| DAY 11 | Sullivan's Dough Breakfast Pizza | Tex-Mex Casserole | Stuffed & Grilled Vegetable Bites | Garlic Bread |
| DAY 12 | Chocolate Pancake Cereal | Spaghetti Squash Casserole | Chicken Alfredo | Keto Bounty Bars |

| | | | | |
|---|---|---|---|---|
| DAY 13 | Frittata with Fresh Spinach | Creamy Chicken, Bacon and Cauliflower Bake | Keto Salad | Funfetti Cookie Bites |
| DAY 14 | Omelet Wrap with Salmon & Avocado | Cauliflower Mash | Cheesy Autumn Mushrooms | Choc-Orange Bliss Balls |
| DAY 15 | Chocolate Pancake Cereal | Easy Tofu Pad Thai | Skillet Pizza | Keto Bounty Bars |
| DAY 16 | Pancakes with Berries and Whipped Cream | Jalapeno Popper Chicken Casserole | Zucchini Bread | Chocolate Chip Cookie Fat Bombs |
| DAY 17 | Mushroom and Cheese Frittat | Easy Tofu Pad Thai | Chicken Garam Masala | Chocolate Chip Cookie Fat Bombs |
| DAY 18 | Keto Cornbread | No Noodle Lasagna | Pimiento Cheese Meatballs | Keto Bounty Bars |
| DAY 19 | Breakfast Sandwich | Stuffed Chicken Breast with Zoodles and Tomato Sauce | Chicken Curry Pie | Cheesecake Fluff |
| DAY 20 | Mushroom and Cheese Frittata | Chicken Wings with Creamy Broccoli | Skillet Pizza | Vanilla Mug Cake |
| DAY 21 | Breakfast Sandwich | Keto Salad | No Noodle Lasagna | Frappuccino Slice |
| DAY 22 | Frittata with Fresh Spinach | Chicken Curry Pie | Taco Pie | French Toast Casserole |
| DAY 23 | Keto Cornbread | Keto Stir Fry | Ginger Lime Chicken | Chocolate Chip Cookie Fat Bombs |
| DAY 24 | Tomato Baked Eggs | Easy Tofu Pad Thai | Skillet Pizza | Chocolate Chaffle Recipe |

| | | | | |
|---|---|---|---|---|
| DAY 25 | Chocolate Pancake Cereal | Keto Salad | Cauliflower Mash | Choc-Orange Bliss Balls |
| DAY 26 | Mexican Egg Roll | Thai Fish Curry | Creamy Chicken, Bacon and Cauliflower Bake | Cheesecake Fluff |
| DAY 27 | Sullivan's Dough Breakfast Pizza | Cauliflower Mash | Taco Pie | Chocolate Peanut Butter Protein Bars |
| DAY 28 | Egg Butter with Smoked Salmon and Avocado | No Noodle Lasagna | Bresaola Plate | Chocolate Mousse |
| DAY 29 | Mushroom and Cheese Frittata | Keto Salad | Easy Chicken Chow Mein | Chocolate Chaffle Recipe |
| DAY 30 | Jill's Cheese-Crusted Omelette | Easy Tofu Pad Thai | Ginger Lime Chicken | Choc-Orange Bliss Balls |

EXTRA: Create your own 1-week meal plan in advance here.

|       | Breakfast | Lunch | Dinner | Snack |
|-------|-----------|-------|--------|-------|
| DAY 1 |           |       |        |       |
| DAY 2 |           |       |        |       |
| DAY 3 |           |       |        |       |
| DAY 4 |           |       |        |       |
| DAY 5 |           |       |        |       |
| DAY 6 |           |       |        |       |
| DAY 7 |           |       |        |       |

## Alphabetical Index Of Recipes

**BREAKFAST RECIPES** ........................................................................................................................... 43
- ALL DAY KETO BREAKFAST ........................................................................................................ 53
- BREAKFAST SANDWICH ............................................................................................................. 54
- CHICKEN CURRY PIE .................................................................................................................... 60
- CHOCOLATE PANCAKE CEREAL ............................................................................................... 57
- CLASSIC BACON AND EGGS ...................................................................................................... 45
- EASY BANANA MUFFINS ............................................................................................................. 58
- EGG BUTTER WITH SMOKED SALMON AND AVOCADO ................................................. 47
- FRITTATA WITH FRESH SPINACH ............................................................................................ 51
- JILL'S CHEESE-CRUSTED OMELETTE ....................................................................................... 44
- KETO CORNBREAD ........................................................................................................................ 55
- MUSHROOM AND CHEESE FRITTATA ..................................................................................... 52
- OMELET WRAP WITH SALMON & AVOCADO ...................................................................... 48
- PANCAKES WITH BERRIES AND WHIPPED CREAM ........................................................... 50
- SCRAMBLED EGGS ........................................................................................................................ 46
- SULLIVAN'S DOUGH BREAKFAST PIZZA ............................................................................... 49
- TOMATO BAKED EGGS ................................................................................................................ 56

**MAIN MEALS** ........................................................................................................................................ 60
- BRESAOLA PLATE .......................................................................................................................... 81
- BUFFALO DRUMSTICKS WITH CHILI AIOLI ......................................................................... 62
- CARAMELIZED ONION AND BACON PORK CHOPS ........................................................... 87
- CAULIFLOWER MASH ................................................................................................................... 76
- CELERY & BLUE CHEESE SOUP ................................................................................................ 91
- CHICKEN ALFREDO ....................................................................................................................... 93
- CHICKEN GARAM MASALA ........................................................................................................ 89
- CHICKEN WINGS WITH CREAMY BROCCOLI ...................................................................... 63
- CRACK CHICKEN ............................................................................................................................ 78
- CREAMY CHICKEN, BACON AND CAULIFLOWER BAKE .................................................. 75
- CRISPY LEMON BAKED CHICKEN THIGHS ........................................................................... 72
- EASY CHICKEN CHOW MEIN ..................................................................................................... 95
- EASY SWEDISH MEATBALLS ...................................................................................................... 94
- EASY TOFU PAD THAI .................................................................................................................. 77
- GINGER LIME CHICKEN ............................................................................................................... 80
- GOAT CHEESEBURGER WITH ZUCCHINI FRIES ................................................................... 84
- HAMBURGER PATTIES WITH CREAMY TOMATO SAUCE AND FRIED CABBAGE ..... 85
- JALAPENO POPPER CHICKEN CASSEROLE ........................................................................... 70
- KETO STIR FRY ................................................................................................................................ 71
- MEXICAN CAULIFLOWER RICE ................................................................................................. 65
- NO NOODLE LASAGNA ................................................................................................................ 79
- OVEN-BAKED PAPRIKA CHICKEN WITH RUTABAGA ....................................................... 86
- PEPPER-CRUSTED BEEF TENDERLOIN WITH HERBED STEAK SAUCE ........................ 64
- PESTO CHICKEN CASSEROLE WITH FETA CHEESE AND OLIVES ................................. 73
- PIMIENTO CHEESE MEATBALLS ............................................................................................... 83
- POT BARBECUE CHICKEN .......................................................................................................... 67

| SKILLET PIZZA | 90 |
|---|---|
| SPAGHETTI SQUASH CASSEROLE | 69 |
| STUFFED CHICKEN BREAST WITH ZOODLES AND TOMATO SAUCE | 74 |
| TACO PIE | 66 |
| TEX-MEX CASSEROLE | 88 |
| THAI FISH CURRY | 92 |
| TURKEY WITH CREAM-CHEESE SAUCE | 82 |

## KETO SNACKS ........ 96

| AVOCADO WITH TAMARI & GINGER DRESSING | 99 |
|---|---|
| BACON BUTTER | 106 |
| CAULIFLOWER TOTS | 103 |
| CHEESY AUTUMN MUSHROOMS | 100 |
| GARLIC BREAD | 107 |
| KETO SALAD | 108 |
| KETO SNACK BOX | 101 |
| MEXICAN EGG ROLL | 102 |
| PROTEIN BALLS | 105 |
| SALAMI CHIPS | 104 |
| STUFFED & GRILLED VEGETABLE BITES | 97 |
| ULTIMATE GUACAMOLE | 98 |

## DESSERTS ........ 109

| BLACKBERRY CHEESECAKE | 122 |
|---|---|
| CHEESECAKE FLUFF | 118 |
| CHOCOLATE CHAFFLE RECIPE | 117 |
| CHOCOLATE CHIP COOKIE FAT BOMBS | 113 |
| CHOCOLATE MOUSSE | 116 |
| CHOCOLATE PEANUT BUTTER PROTEIN BARS | 114 |
| CHOC-ORANGE BLISS BALLS | 111 |
| FRAPPUCCINO SLICE | 110 |
| FRENCH TOAST CASSEROLE | 120 |
| FUNFETTI COOKIE BITES | 121 |
| KETO BOUNTY BARS | 112 |
| PUMPKIN PANCAKES | 119 |
| STRAWBERRY CHEESECAKE | 123 |

# PART 4

## The Keto Diet Journal

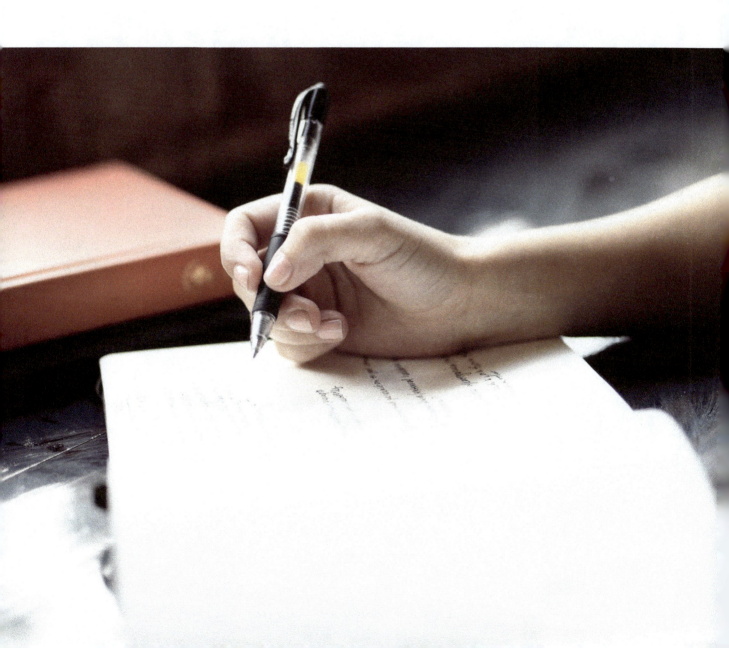

# Progress Tracker

*"It took more than a day to put it on. It will take more than a day to take it off."*

| What to track | WEEK 1 | WEEK2 | WEEK 3 | WEEK 4 |
|---|---|---|---|---|
| Weight | | | | |
| Chest | | | | |
| Hips | | | | |
| L/R arm | | | | |
| L/R thigh | | | | |

## My weight goal is:

# MONTHLY PROGRESS TRACKER

| MON | TUE | WED | THU | FRI | SAT | SUN |
|---|---|---|---|---|---|---|
|  |  |  |  |  |  |  |
|  |  |  |  |  |  |  |
|  |  |  |  |  |  |  |
|  |  |  |  |  |  |  |
|  |  |  |  |  |  |  |

WEIGHT LOSS MILESTONE TRACKER

_____
_____
_____
_____

CHEAT DAY TRACKER

_____
_____
_____
_____

WEEKLY DIET SUCCESS TRACKER & NOTES

_____
_____
_____
_____

# YEARLY DAY TRACKER

|    | JAN | FEB | MAR | APR | MAY | JUN | JUL | AUG | SEP | OCT | NOV | DEC |
|----|-----|-----|-----|-----|-----|-----|-----|-----|-----|-----|-----|-----|
| 1  |     |     |     |     |     |     |     |     |     |     |     |     |
| 2  |     |     |     |     |     |     |     |     |     |     |     |     |
| 3  |     |     |     |     |     |     |     |     |     |     |     |     |
| 4  |     |     |     |     |     |     |     |     |     |     |     |     |
| 5  |     |     |     |     |     |     |     |     |     |     |     |     |
| 6  |     |     |     |     |     |     |     |     |     |     |     |     |
| 7  |     |     |     |     |     |     |     |     |     |     |     |     |
| 8  |     |     |     |     |     |     |     |     |     |     |     |     |
| 9  |     |     |     |     |     |     |     |     |     |     |     |     |
| 10 |     |     |     |     |     |     |     |     |     |     |     |     |
| 11 |     |     |     |     |     |     |     |     |     |     |     |     |
| 12 |     |     |     |     |     |     |     |     |     |     |     |     |
| 13 |     |     |     |     |     |     |     |     |     |     |     |     |
| 14 |     |     |     |     |     |     |     |     |     |     |     |     |
| 15 |     |     |     |     |     |     |     |     |     |     |     |     |
| 16 |     |     |     |     |     |     |     |     |     |     |     |     |
| 17 |     |     |     |     |     |     |     |     |     |     |     |     |
| 18 |     |     |     |     |     |     |     |     |     |     |     |     |
| 19 |     |     |     |     |     |     |     |     |     |     |     |     |
| 20 |     |     |     |     |     |     |     |     |     |     |     |     |
| 21 |     |     |     |     |     |     |     |     |     |     |     |     |
| 22 |     |     |     |     |     |     |     |     |     |     |     |     |
| 23 |     |     |     |     |     |     |     |     |     |     |     |     |
| 24 |     |     |     |     |     |     |     |     |     |     |     |     |
| 25 |     |     |     |     |     |     |     |     |     |     |     |     |
| 26 |     |     |     |     |     |     |     |     |     |     |     |     |
| 27 |     |     |     |     |     |     |     |     |     |     |     |     |
| 28 |     |     |     |     |     |     |     |     |     |     |     |     |
| 29 |     |     |     |     |     |     |     |     |     |     |     |     |
| 30 |     |     |     |     |     |     |     |     |     |     |     |     |
| 31 |     |     |     |     |     |     |     |     |     |     |     |     |

*Color in the days that you were in ketosis to keep track of your weight loss progress.*

Notes

_____

_____

_____

_____

_____

_____

_____

_____

_____

_____

_____

_____

_____

_____

_____

# Notes/Observations:

# day 01

Date _____

| | | Cals | Carbs | Fats | Pro |
|---|---|---|---|---|---|
| Breakfast | | | | | |
| Lunch | | | | | |
| Dinner | | | | | |
| Snack | | | | | |

### Today's macro total

| Cals | Carbs | Fats | Pro |
|---|---|---|---|
| | | | |

### Today's notes

_____

_____

_____

## Shopping List

## Hydration

 X _____

## Today I feel...

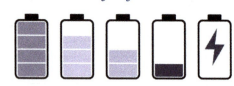

## Exercise

| Type | Mins/Hrs |
|---|---|
| | |

# day 02

Date _____

|  | | Cals | Carbs | Fats | Pro |
|---|---|---|---|---|---|
| Breakfast | | | | | |
| Lunch | | Cals | Carbs | Fats | Pro |
| | | | | | |
| Dinner | | Cals | Carbs | Fats | Pro |
| | | | | | |
| Snack | | Cals | Carbs | Fats | Pro |
| | | | | | |

## Shopping List

## Hydration

 X _____

## Today I feel...

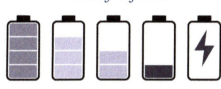

## Today's macro total

| Cals | Carbs | Fats | Pro |
|---|---|---|---|
| | | | |

## Exercise

| Type | Mins/Hrs |
|---|---|
| | |
| | |

## Today's notes

_____

_____

_____

# day 03

Date _____

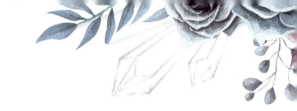

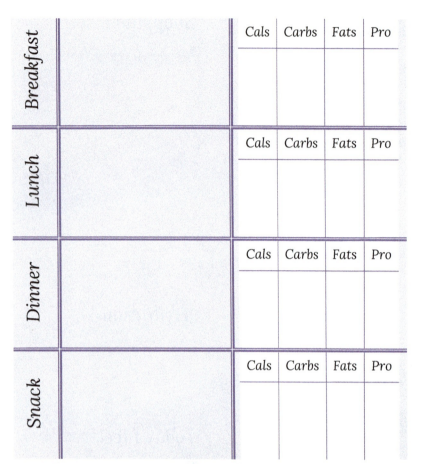

## Shopping List

## Hydration

 X _____

## Today I feel...

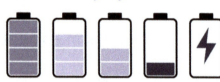

## Today's macro total

| Cals | Carbs | Fats | Pro |
|---|---|---|---|
|  |  |  |  |

## Exercise

| Type | Mins/Hrs |
|---|---|
|  |  |

## Today's notes

_____
_____
_____

# day 04

Date _____

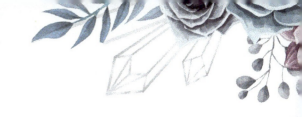

| | | Cals | Carbs | Fats | Pro |
|---|---|---|---|---|---|
| Breakfast | | | | | |
| Lunch | | | | | |
| Dinner | | | | | |
| Snack | | | | | |

## Shopping List

## Hydration

 X _____

## Today I feel...

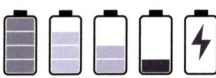

## Today's macro total

| Cals | Carbs | Fats | Pro |
|---|---|---|---|
| | | | |

## Exercise

| Type | Mins/Hrs |
|---|---|
| | |

## Today's notes

_____
_____
_____

# day 05

Date _____

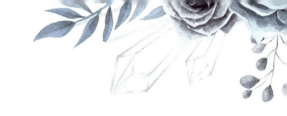

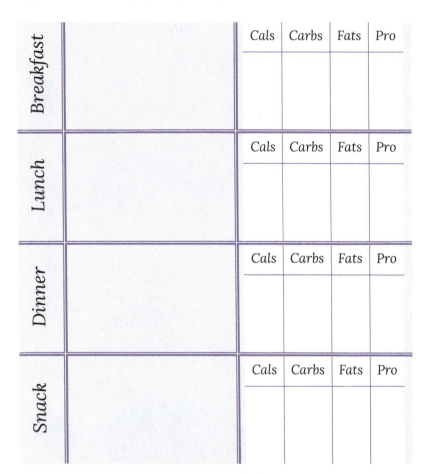

## Shopping List

## Hydration

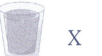 X _____

## Today I feel...

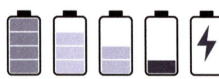

## Today's macro total

| Cals | Carbs | Fats | Pro |
|------|-------|------|-----|
|      |       |      |     |

## Exercise

| Type | Mins/Hrs |
|------|----------|
|      |          |

## Today's notes

_____
_____
_____

# day 06

Date _____

| | | Cals | Carbs | Fats | Pro |
|---|---|---|---|---|---|
| Breakfast | | | | | |
| Lunch | | | | | |
| Dinner | | | | | |
| Snack | | | | | |

## Shopping List

## Hydration

 X _____

## Today's macro total

| Cals | Carbs | Fats | Pro |
|---|---|---|---|
| | | | |

## Today I feel...

## Today's notes

_____
_____
_____

## Exercise

| Type | Mins/Hrs |
|---|---|
| | |

# day 07

Date _____

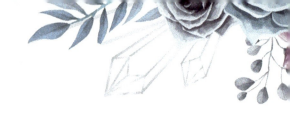

| | | Cals | Carbs | Fats | Pro |
|---|---|---|---|---|---|
| Breakfast | | | | | |
| Lunch | | | | | |
| Dinner | | | | | |
| Snack | | | | | |

## Today's macro total

| Cals | Carbs | Fats | Pro |
|---|---|---|---|
| | | | |

## Today's notes

_____
_____
_____

## Shopping List

## Hydration

  X  _____

## Today I feel...

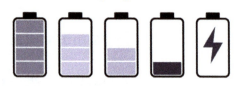

## Exercise

| Type | Mins/Hrs |
|---|---|
| | |

# day 08

Date _____

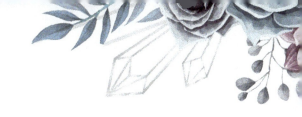

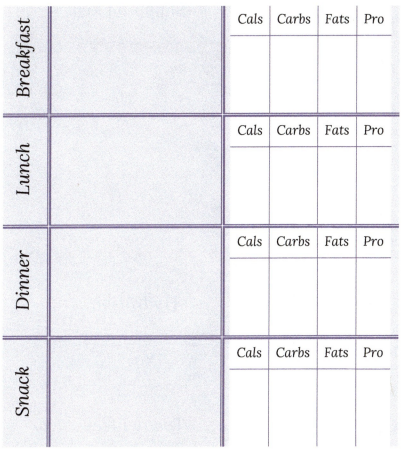

## Shopping List

## Hydration

 X _____

## Today I feel...

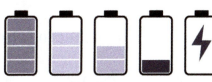

## Today's macro total

| Cals | Carbs | Fats | Pro |
|------|-------|------|-----|
|      |       |      |     |

## Exercise

| Type | Mins/Hrs |
|------|----------|
|      |          |

## Today's notes

_____
_____
_____

# day 09

Date _____

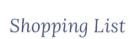

|  | | Cals | Carbs | Fats | Pro |
|---|---|---|---|---|---|
| Breakfast | | | | | |
| Lunch | | | | | |
| Dinner | | | | | |
| Snack | | | | | |

## Shopping List

## Hydration

 X _____

## Today's macro total

| Cals | Carbs | Fats | Pro |
|---|---|---|---|
| | | | |

## Today I feel…

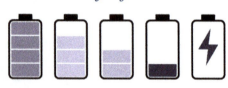

## Exercise

| Type | Mins/Hrs |
|---|---|
| | |

## Today's notes

_____
_____
_____

# day 10

Date _____

|  | | Cals | Carbs | Fats | Pro |
|---|---|---|---|---|---|
| Breakfast | | | | | |
| Lunch | | | | | |
| Dinner | | | | | |
| Snack | | | | | |

### Today's macro total

| Cals | Carbs | Fats | Pro |
|---|---|---|---|
| | | | |

### Today's notes

_____
_____
_____

## Shopping List

## Hydration

 X _____

## Today I feel...

## Exercise

| Type | Mins/Hrs |
|---|---|
| | |

# day 11

Date  _____

| | | Cals | Carbs | Fats | Pro |
|---|---|---|---|---|---|
| Breakfast | | | | | |
| Lunch | | | | | |
| Dinner | | | | | |
| Snack | | | | | |

### Today's macro total

| Cals | Carbs | Fats | Pro |
|---|---|---|---|
| | | | |

### Today's notes

_____

_____

_____

## Shopping List

## Hydration

  X  _____

## Today I feel...

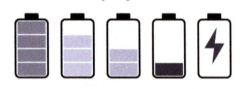

## Exercise

| Type | Mins/Hrs |
|---|---|
| | |

# day 12

Date _____

| | | Cals | Carbs | Fats | Pro |
|---|---|---|---|---|---|
| Breakfast | | | | | |
| Lunch | | | | | |
| Dinner | | | | | |
| Snack | | | | | |

## Shopping List

## Hydration

 X _____

## Today I feel...

## Today's macro total

| Cals | Carbs | Fats | Pro |
|---|---|---|---|
| | | | |

## Today's notes

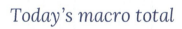

## Exercise

| Type | Mins/Hrs |
|---|---|
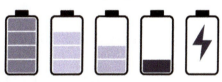

# day 13

Date _____

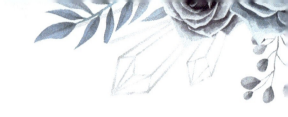

|  |  | Cals | Carbs | Fats | Pro |
|---|---|---|---|---|---|
| Breakfast |  |  |  |  |  |
| Lunch |  |  |  |  |  |
| Dinner |  |  |  |  |  |
| Snack |  |  |  |  |  |

## Shopping List

## Hydration

 X _____

## Today I feel...

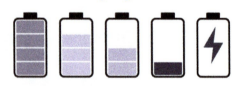

## Today's macro total

| Cals | Carbs | Fats | Pro |
|---|---|---|---|
|  |  |  |  |

## Today's notes

_____
_____
_____

## Exercise

| Type | Mins/Hrs |
|---|---|
|  |  |

# day 14

Date _____

| Breakfast | | Cals | Carbs | Fats | Pro |
|---|---|---|---|---|---|
| Lunch | | Cals | Carbs | Fats | Pro |
| Dinner | | Cals | Carbs | Fats | Pro |
| Snack | | Cals | Carbs | Fats | Pro |

## Shopping List

## Hydration

 X _____

## Today I feel...

## Today's macro total

| Cals | Carbs | Fats | Pro |
|---|---|---|---|
| | | | |

## Exercise

| Type | Mins/Hrs |
|---|---|
| | |

## Today's notes

_____
_____
_____

# day 15

Date _____

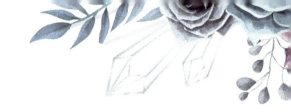

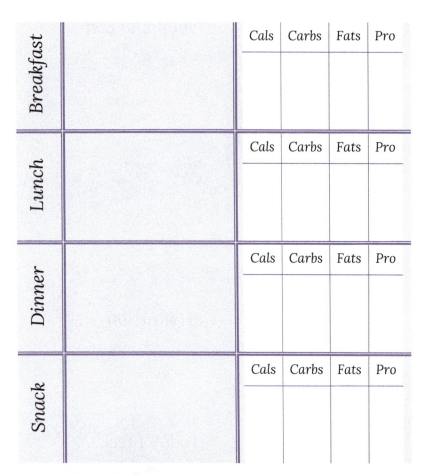

| | Cals | Carbs | Fats | Pro |
|---|---|---|---|---|
| Breakfast | | | | |
| Lunch | | | | |
| Dinner | | | | |
| Snack | | | | |

## Shopping List

## Hydration

 X _____

## Today I feel...

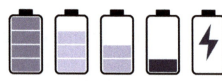

### Today's macro total

| Cals | Carbs | Fats | Pro |
|---|---|---|---|
| | | | |

### Today's notes

_____
_____
_____

### Exercise

| Type | Mins/Hrs |
|---|---|
| | |

# day 16

Date _____

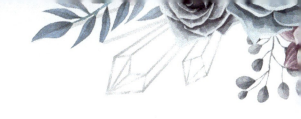

| | | Cals | Carbs | Fats | Pro |
|---|---|---|---|---|---|
| Breakfast | | | | | |
| Lunch | | | | | |
| Dinner | | | | | |
| Snack | | | | | |

## Shopping List

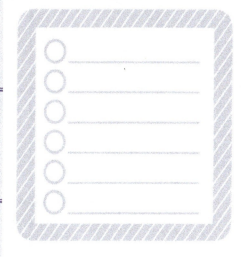

## Hydration

 X _____

## Today's macro total

| Cals | Carbs | Fats | Pro |
|---|---|---|---|
| | | | |

## Today I feel...

## Exercise

| Type | Mins/Hrs |
|---|---|
| | |

## Today's notes

_____
_____
_____

# day 17

Date _____

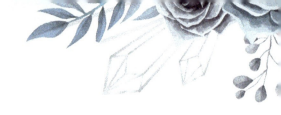

|  | | Cals | Carbs | Fats | Pro |
|---|---|---|---|---|---|
| Breakfast | | | | | |
| Lunch | | | | | |
| Dinner | | | | | |
| Snack | | | | | |

## Today's macro total

| Cals | Carbs | Fats | Pro |
|---|---|---|---|
| | | | |

## Today's notes

_____
_____
_____

## Shopping List

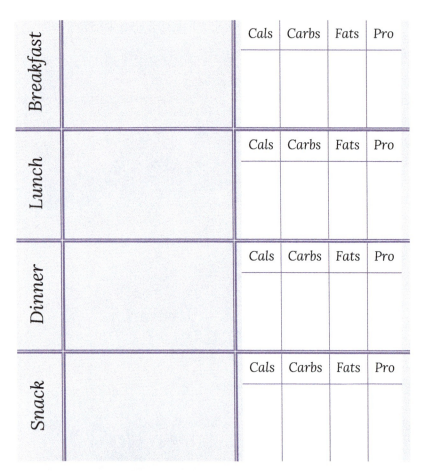

## Hydration

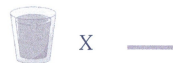 X _____

## Today I feel...

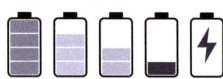

## Exercise

| Type | Mins/Hrs |
|---|---|
| | |

# day 18

Date _____

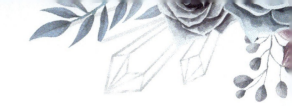

|  | | Cals | Carbs | Fats | Pro |
|---|---|---|---|---|---|
| Breakfast | | | | | |
| Lunch | | | | | |
| Dinner | | | | | |
| Snack | | | | | |

## Shopping List

## Hydration

 X _____

## Today's macro total

| Cals | Carbs | Fats | Pro |
|---|---|---|---|
| | | | |

## Today I feel...

## Today's notes

_____

_____

_____

## Exercise

| Type | Mins/Hrs |
|---|---|
| | |

# day 19

Date _____

| | | Cals | Carbs | Fats | Pro |
|---|---|---|---|---|---|
| Breakfast | | | | | |
| Lunch | | | | | |
| Dinner | | | | | |
| Snack | | | | | |

### Today's macro total

| Cals | Carbs | Fats | Pro |
|---|---|---|---|
| | | | |

### Today's notes

_____
_____
_____

### Shopping List

### Hydration

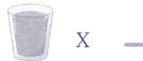 X _____

### Today I feel...

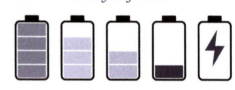

### Exercise

| Type | Mins/Hrs |
|---|---|
| | |

day 20

Date _____

|  | | Cals | Carbs | Fats | Pro |
|---|---|---|---|---|---|
| Breakfast | | | | | |
| Lunch | | | | | |
| Dinner | | | | | |
| Snack | | | | | |

Shopping List

Hydration

 X _____

Today I feel...

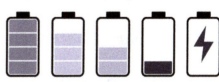

### Today's macro total

| Cals | Carbs | Fats | Pro |
|---|---|---|---|
| | | | |

### Exercise

| Type | Mins/Hrs |
|---|---|
| | |

### Today's notes

_____
_____
_____

# day 21

Date _____

|  | | Cals | Carbs | Fats | Pro |
|---|---|---|---|---|---|
| Breakfast | | | | | |
| Lunch | | | | | |
| Dinner | | | | | |
| Snack | | | | | |

## Today's macro total

| Cals | Carbs | Fats | Pro |
|---|---|---|---|
| | | | |

## Today's notes

_____

_____

_____

## Shopping List

## Hydration

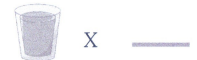 X _____

## Today I feel...

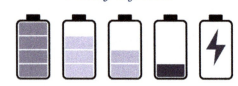

## Exercise

| Type | Mins/Hrs |
|---|---|
| | |

# day 22

Date _____

|  | | Cals | Carbs | Fats | Pro |
|---|---|---|---|---|---|
| Breakfast | | | | | |
| Lunch | | | | | |
| Dinner | | | | | |
| Snack | | | | | |

## Shopping List

## Hydration

 X _____

## Today's macro total

| Cals | Carbs | Fats | Pro |
|---|---|---|---|
| | | | |

## Today I feel...

## Exercise

| Type | Mins/Hrs |
|---|---|
| | |

## Today's notes

_____
_____
_____

# day 23

Date _____

| | | Cals | Carbs | Fats | Pro |
|---|---|---|---|---|---|
| Breakfast | | | | | |
| Lunch | | | | | |
| Dinner | | | | | |
| Snack | | | | | |

## Shopping List

## Hydration

 X _____

## Today I feel...

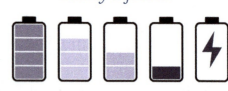

## Today's macro total

| Cals | Carbs | Fats | Pro |
|---|---|---|---|
| | | | |

## Exercise

| Type | Mins/Hrs |
|---|---|
| | |

## Today's notes

_____

_____

_____

# day 24

Date _____

| | | Cals | Carbs | Fats | Pro |
|---|---|---|---|---|---|
| Breakfast | | | | | |
| Lunch | | | | | |
| Dinner | | | | | |
| Snack | | | | | |

## Today's macro total

| Cals | Carbs | Fats | Pro |
|---|---|---|---|
| | | | |

## Today's notes

_____
_____
_____

### Shopping List

### Hydration

 X _____

### Today I feel...

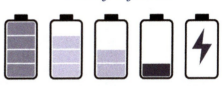

### Exercise

| Type | Mins/Hrs |
|---|---|
| | |

# day 25

Date _____

|  | | Cals | Carbs | Fats | Pro |
|---|---|---|---|---|---|
| Breakfast | | | | | |
| Lunch | | | | | |
| Dinner | | | | | |
| Snack | | | | | |

## Today's macro total

| Cals | Carbs | Fats | Pro |
|---|---|---|---|
| | | | |

### Today's notes

_____
_____
_____

## Shopping List

## Hydration

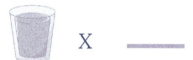

X _____

## Today I feel...

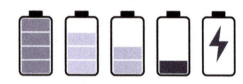

## Exercise

| Type | Mins/Hrs |
|---|---|
| | |

# day 26

Date _____

| | | Cals | Carbs | Fats | Pro |
|---|---|---|---|---|---|
| Breakfast | | | | | |
| Lunch | | | | | |
| Dinner | | | | | |
| Snack | | | | | |

## Shopping List

## Hydration

 X _____

## Today's macro total

| Cals | Carbs | Fats | Pro |
|---|---|---|---|
| | | | |

## Today I feel...

## Exercise

| Type | Mins/Hrs |
|---|---|
| | |

## Today's notes

_____

_____

_____

# day 27

Date _____

| | | Cals | Carbs | Fats | Pro |
|---|---|---|---|---|---|
| Breakfast | | | | | |
| Lunch | | Cals | Carbs | Fats | Pro |
| | | | | | |
| Dinner | | Cals | Carbs | Fats | Pro |
| | | | | | |
| Snack | | Cals | Carbs | Fats | Pro |
| | | | | | |

## Today's macro total

| Cals | Carbs | Fats | Pro |
|---|---|---|---|
| | | | |

## Today's notes

_____
_____
_____

## Shopping List

## Hydration

 X _____

## Today I feel...

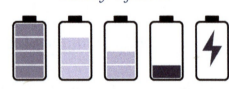

## Exercise

| Type | Mins/Hrs |
|---|---|
| | |

# day 28

Date _____

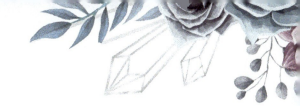

|  | | Cals | Carbs | Fats | Pro |
|---|---|---|---|---|---|
| Breakfast | | | | | |
| Lunch | | | | | |
| Dinner | | | | | |
| Snack | | | | | |

## Shopping List

## Hydration

 X _____

## Today's macro total

| Cals | Carbs | Fats | Pro |
|---|---|---|---|
| | | | |

## Today I feel...

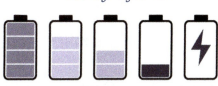

## Exercise

| Type | Mins/Hrs |
|---|---|
| | |

## Today's notes

_____
_____
_____

# day 29

Date _____

| | | Cals | Carbs | Fats | Pro |
|---|---|---|---|---|---|
| Breakfast | | | | | |
| Lunch | | | | | |
| Dinner | | | | | |
| Snack | | | | | |

## Today's macro total

| Cals | Carbs | Fats | Pro |
|---|---|---|---|
| | | | |

## Today's notes

_____
_____
_____

## Shopping List

## Hydration

 X _____

## Today I feel...

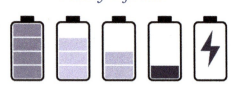

## Exercise

| Type | Mins/Hrs |
|---|---|
| | |

# day 30

Date _____

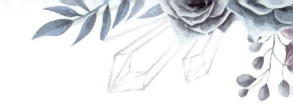

| | | Cals | Carbs | Fats | Pro |
|---|---|---|---|---|---|
| Breakfast | | | | | |
| Lunch | | | | | |
| Dinner | | | | | |
| Snack | | | | | |

## Shopping List

## Hydration

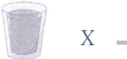  X _____

## Today's macro total

| Cals | Carbs | Fats | Pro |
|---|---|---|---|
| | | | |

## Today I feel...

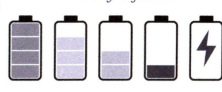

## Exercise

| Type | Mins/Hrs |
|---|---|
| | |

## Today's notes

_____
_____
_____

Date: _____

## My Weight Goal Was:

_____

## My Final Weight Is:

_____

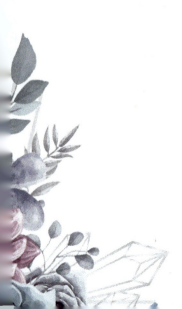

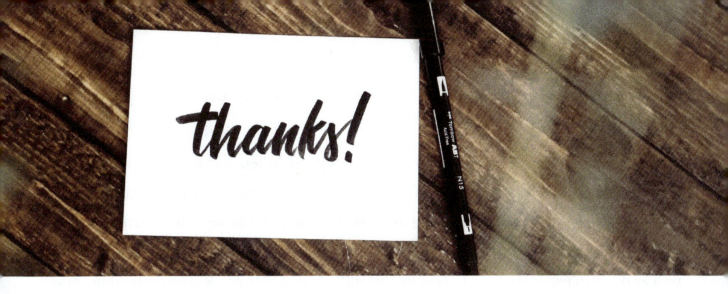

## Final Words

Thank you for reading this book!

This is the 5th book I've written since 2016. It took me months to write this one, partly because I am a full-time mom and nutritionist. The main reason, however, is that I decided to challenge myself even more this time.

My goal for this guide was to put very complex and technical concepts in the simplest way, so as to make it readable for everyone.

To do so, I accurately selected what I believe are the most useful and effective pieces of advice for you. In my 20 years+ of professional experience I've had the amazing chance to deal with hundreds of people of all ages, gender, and personality, and it inevitably has some reflections on my writings.

I don't like to call myself an author, yet I have to admit that I learned a lot while writing books over the past few years. In fact, what I got from those past publications was validation from readers who enjoyed my work and encouraged me to keep writing.

I always value the opinion of readers because I do believe that reviews are a great way to give someone credit for all the work done, and, plus, I love reading them!

It's a fact that readers do the same before purchasing books; that's why I give special importance to reviews and I feel bad when I get a critical one.

Anyway, I hope you keep in mind that I am a self-published author, without the huge possibilities that publishing houses have (such as proofreading, special formatting and so on...). However, I hope I accomplished at least the goal I had in my mind - which was to provide you precious information about intermittent fasting, based on scientific studies as well as my own experience, and, most importantly, I hope that you learned something new and will act on it to change your life.

Special thanks go to my family, in particular to my beloved husband and my two little daughters, who read this book before than anyone else. I got great feedbacks from them and I am elated about that, even though I think they are a little bit biased!

After all, they have seen me when at nights, after exhausting workdays, I locked myself up in the study room, writing and organizing this guide in the best possible way.

I hope you will keep that in mind too and consider using some seconds of your precious time to leave a review on this book. I keep harping on this because it is just so important to me, especially in a more and more crowded and difficult world of book publishing.

I will be GRATEFUL for each one of you.

P.S. I'm a nutritionist, I am a mom, I am a woman but above all... I am a human being. An immaculate work is far from reality, especially when you write alone.

So, please, if you wish to report any typos or inaccuracies you encountered in this guide, or have something to complain about, email me directly at leanneaxedoctor@nutritionist.com. I always take into account any request and will make my best to meet the requests.

*Dr. Leanne Axe*

CPSIA information can be obtained
at www.ICGtesting.com
Printed in the USA
LVHW060530130121
676353LV00005B/174